NUTRITION AND DIET RESEARCH PROGRESS

PLANTS FOR WEIGHT LOSS – MYTH AND REALITY

NUTRITION AND DIET
RESEARCH PROGRESS

Additional books and e-books in this series can be found on Nova's website under the Series tab.

NUTRITION AND DIET RESEARCH PROGRESS

PLANTS FOR WEIGHT LOSS – MYTH AND REALITY

ALEXANDER V. SIROTKIN

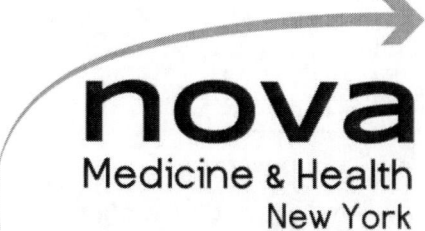

Copyright © 2020 by Nova Science Publishers, Inc.

All rights reserved. No part of this book may be reproduced, stored in a retrieval system or transmitted in any form or by any means: electronic, electrostatic, magnetic, tape, mechanical photocopying, recording or otherwise without the written permission of the Publisher.

We have partnered with Copyright Clearance Center to make it easy for you to obtain permissions to reuse content from this publication. Simply navigate to this publication's page on Nova's website and locate the "Get Permission" button below the title description. This button is linked directly to the title's permission page on copyright.com. Alternatively, you can visit copyright.com and search by title, ISBN, or ISSN.

For further questions about using the service on copyright.com, please contact:
Copyright Clearance Center
Phone: +1-(978) 750-8400   Fax: +1-(978) 750-4470   E-mail: info@copyright.com.

NOTICE TO THE READER

The Publisher has taken reasonable care in the preparation of this book, but makes no expressed or implied warranty of any kind and assumes no responsibility for any errors or omissions. No liability is assumed for incidental or consequential damages in connection with or arising out of information contained in this book. The Publisher shall not be liable for any special, consequential, or exemplary damages resulting, in whole or in part, from the readers' use of, or reliance upon, this material. Any parts of this book based on government reports are so indicated and copyright is claimed for those parts to the extent applicable to compilations of such works.

Independent verification should be sought for any data, advice or recommendations contained in this book. In addition, no responsibility is assumed by the Publisher for any injury and/or damage to persons or property arising from any methods, products, instructions, ideas or otherwise contained in this publication.

This publication is designed to provide accurate and authoritative information with regard to the subject matter covered herein. It is sold with the clear understanding that the Publisher is not engaged in rendering legal or any other professional services. If legal or any other expert assistance is required, the services of a competent person should be sought. FROM A DECLARATION OF PARTICIPANTS JOINTLY ADOPTED BY A COMMITTEE OF THE AMERICAN BAR ASSOCIATION AND A COMMITTEE OF PUBLISHERS.

Additional color graphics may be available in the e-book version of this book.

Library of Congress Cataloging-in-Publication Data

Names: Sirotkin, Alexander V., author.
Title: Plants for weight loss : myth and reality / Alexander V. Sirotkin.
Description: New York : Nova Science Publishers, [2021] | Series: Nutrition and diet research progress | Includes bibliographical references and index. | Summary: "This is a unique book which critically summarizes the current scientific knowledge concerning manifestations, mechanisms, consequences and prevention of dysfunctions of metabolism of fat, as well as the main known functional food and medicinal plants which can be and which cannot be used for prevention and treatment of obesity. The provenance, biologically active molecules, positive and adverse side-effects on health, influence on obesity and potential applicability of tea, chicory, Garcinia cambogia, Hoodia gordonii, chia, Irvingia gabonensis, apple cider vinegar, coffee, konjac/glucomannan, flaxseed, mulberry, oat, sweet and hot peppers, carob, cinnamon, plum, Cissus quadrangularis, Stevia rebaudiana, Yacon and ginger are described in details. In addition, less-known plants and plant molecules, as well as their combinations considered applicable for obesity treatments, are listed. It is demonstrated that more than half of the plant-based anti-obesity products available on the market are not properly clinically tested, or such tests, when performed, provided negative results. In addition, the author provides the reader with some practical advices and tips to combat obesity with healthy lifestyle. This book combines deep scientific analysis of physiological processes and popular form of their description. Such form enables to use this knowledge and advices for scientists, doctors, producers, distributors and consumers of functional food and medicinal plants, as well as for the common readers interested in healthy nutrition and life style"-- Provided by publisher. Identifiers: LCCN 2020043026 (print) | LCCN 2020043027 (ebook) | ISBN 9781536187007 (softcover) | ISBN 9781536187472 (adobe pdf)
Subjects: LCSH: Reducing diets. | Medicinal plants. | Functional foods.
Classification: LCC RM222.2 S5575 2021 (print) | LCC RM222.2 (ebook) | DDC 615.3/21--dc23
LC record available at https://lccn.loc.gov/2020043026
LC ebook record available at https://lccn.loc.gov/2020043027

Published by Nova Science Publishers, Inc. † New York

CONTENTS

Preface		**ix**
Chapter 1	Introduction	**1**
	1.1. What Is This Book About?	1
	1.2. What Influences Our Weight, Shape and Health?	4
Chapter 2	Selected Plants and Their Molecules, Which Can Impact Fat Stores	**19**
	2.1. Introduction: How Can Plants Help in Weight Loss?	19
	2.2. Apple Cider Vinegar	20
	2.3. Carob (Ceratonia siliqua L.).	23
	2.4. Coffee (Coffea arabica and Coffea canephora)	26
	2.5. Cinnamon	31
	2.6. Chia (Salvia hispanica L.)	34
	2.7. Chicory (Cichorium intybus L.) and Its Molecule Inulin	36
	2.8. Flaxseed (Linum usitatissimum L.)	41
	2.9. Garcinia cambogia	45
	2.10. Ginger (Zingiber zerumbet L.)	48

	2.11. Hoodia gorgonii	52
	2.12. Irvingia gabonensis	55
	2.13. Konjac (Amorphophallus konjac K. Koch) and Its Molecule Glucomannan	58
	2.14. Mulberry (Morus spp.)	61
	2.15. Oat (Avena sativa L.)	66
	2.16. Peppers (Capsicum spp.)	70
	2.17. Plum (Prunus domestica L.)	75
	2.18. Stevia/Candyleaf (Stevia rebaudiana Bertoni)	78
	2.19. Tea (Camelia sinensis L.)	82
	2.20. Veld grape (Cissus quadrangularis L.)	87
	2.21. Yacón (Smallanthus sonchifolius Poepp.)	90
	2.22. Yerba Maté (Ilex paraguariensis A.-St.-Hil)	93
	2.23. Less Popular Plant-Based Weight Loss Supplements	96
Chapter 3	Which Plants Are Best for Weight Loss and What Does It Depend On?	**103**
Chapter 4	Combinations of Individual Plant Molecules	**107**
	4.1. Similar Effects of Individual Plant Molecules	107
	4.2. Possible Interactions of the Individual Plant Molecules	109
	4.3. Possible Combinations of Plant Molecules	109
Chapter 5	Some Myths About the Effect of Plant Molecules Influencing Body Weight	**113**
	5.1. Examples of Plant Molecules Undeservedly Believed to Facilitate Obesity	113
	5.2. Examples of Plant Molecules Mistakenly Assumed to Help In Weight Loss	114
Chapter 6	Conclusion: What We Learned	**117**
Summary		**123**

Bibliography **125**
    References *125*
    Website Links *170*

About the Author **175**

Index **177**

PREFACE

This is a unique book which critically summarizes the current scientific knowledge concerning manifestations, mechanisms, consequences and prevention of dysfunctions of metabolism of fat, as well as the main known functional food and medicinal plants which can be and which cannot be used for prevention and treatment of obesity. The provenance, biologically active molecules, positive and adverse side-effects on health, influence on obesity and potential applicability of tea, chicory, *Garcinia cambogia*, *Hoodia gordonii*, chia, *Irvingia gabonensis*, apple cider vinegar, coffee, konjac/glucomannan, flaxseed, mulberry, oat, sweet and hot peppers, carob, cinnamon, plum, *Cissus quadrangularis*, *Stevia rebaudiana*, Yacon and ginger are described in details. In addition, less-known plants and plant molecules, as well as their combinations considered applicable for obesity treatments, are listed. It is demonstrated that more than half of the plant-based anti-obesity products available on the market are not properly clinically tested, or such tests, when performed, provided negative results. In addition, the author provides the reader with some practical advices and tips to combat obesity with healthy lifestyle. This book combines deep scientific analysis of physiological processes and popular form of their description. Such form enables to use this knowledge and advices for scientists, doctors, producers, distributers and consumers of functional food and medicinal plants, as well as for the common readers interested in healthy nutrition and life style.

Chapter 1

INTRODUCTION

"All food is functional, but some food is more functional than others."
Peter Gerely, European Platform for Functional Food

1.1. WHAT IS THIS BOOK ABOUT?

It is paradoxical that achieving the human dream – elimination of poverty and hard manual labour, along with acquiring sufficient leisure time – endangers the health, quality of life, and longevity of people. World's leading cause of death are diseases related to metabolic dysfunctions. The most significant in this aspect is overweight, which affects 1.9 billion of people around the world, of whom 650 million are obese (Haider and Larose, 2019). In the last 40 years, the number of obese people in the world has tripled and thus we can speak of obesity pandemic (Atawia et al., 2019). Obesity and overweight can facilitate diabetes, cause inflammations, cardiovascular and reproductive diseases as well as cancer (Skrypnik et al., 2017, Sung et al., 2018). In addition to these health risks, they are a cause of mobility issues, as well as problems in social and sexual relationships. They lower self-esteem and the overall quality of life. They also lead to considerable economic losses. Health care concerning patients with obesity incurs at least 25% higher expenditures and causes losses of 1–3.6% of the gross domestic product of a country (Mohamed et al., 2014).

Prevention and treatment of metabolic disorders requires a search for methods to reduce calorie intake and storing and, on the other hand, to increase their burning. With minimal effects on the overall quality of nutrition and life, naturally. One of the options to achieve this goal is to introduce into diet foods with added value (sometimes called functional foods), which reduce fat accumulation and weight in a natural way (Sung et al., 2018).

A current problem of the humankind is also the opposite extreme – malnutrition. In 2018, in 53 countries approximately 113 million people suffered from hunger. Another 143 millions of inhabitants of 42 countries are approaching acute hunger (https://www.hlavnespravy.sk/krutym-hladom-trpi-vo-svete-podla-statistiky-viac-ako-100-milionov-ludi/1726018). The number of cases of malnutrition due to psychosomatic causes – people suffering from *anorexia nervosa* – is growing. This mental disorder affects approximately 1% of women worldwide. Among mental disorders, anorexia is the leading cause of death (Steinglass and Walsh, 2016). The problem of hunger is being solved through development of agriculture rather than medicine. Pharmacological and psychiatric treatment of anorexia has not been very successful as of yet. Treatment of issues connected to malnutrition through medicinal plants is possible in theory, but there is a lack of the corresponding data in the literature. Therefore, this book will not examine this topic. We will focus on treatment and prevention of overweight and obesity using plants and their active molecules.

Prevention and treatment of diseases using natural products of plant origin have always been the foundation of folk and oriental medicine. Nowadays, they are experiencing a renaissance and their popularity is growing even in the official medicine and self-treatment. However, most people get their information and ideas primarily from their family, friends, social media and marketing campaigns. Marketers have, of course, a vested interest in the demand for their "miraculous" products. Therefore, they occasionally take advantage of the metabolic issues plaguing people and the increased interest in products made of medicinal plants. Many of the preparations they offer have not been scientifically and clinically tested. Or, when such tests were carried out, they even demonstrated their lack of effect. Unfortunately, the public rarely has an access to verified scientific data.

This publication aspires to be a scientific monograph, which contains a critical overview of validated and non-validated knowledge. At the same time, it wants to be comprehensible, interesting and useful even for a reader without a scientific background. It offers a review of the most recent (published primarily after 2000) scientific publications in the databases of scientific publications MedLine and SCOPUS on the topics of manifestation, mechanisms, consequences and prevention of dysfunctions of the lipid metabolism. It includes also practical advice on what to do and not do against these dysfunctions. At the same time, the book contains an overview of plant preparations most often used to facilitate weight loss. These plants and plant molecules are tea, chicory/inulin, *Garcinia cambogia*, *Hoodia gordinii*, chia, *Irvingia gabonensis*, apple cider vinegar, coffee, konjak/glucomannan, flax, mulberry, oat, sweet and hot peppers, carob, cinnamon, plum, veld grape, Stevia, Yacón, Yerba Maté, and ginger. Each of them is briefly described in regards to its provenance, biologically active molecules, their positive effect on health, and their effect on obesity. Mentioned are also any adverse side-effects, if such exist. In this book you will find also some recommendations for the use of these substances in reduction of weight and obesity. Included is also a list of less popular plants with similar effects. Each piece of information is supplemented with references to the corresponding sources, which enables the reader to verify it. In this monograph, we tried to review these data critically and based on that evaluation, to provide suggestions for use of these plants and preparations made of them. You will find also the best-known combinations of the plant products with positive therapeutic effect in obese patients. Discussed are also the most common myths about plants' ability to increase or reduce the fat stores in humans. Our knowledge and suggestions are only in regards to the biomedicinal characteristics and not the production, cost, or sensory aspects of the products. We hope that this information and advice will help the lay public as well as experts to correctly select plant preparations and determine their dosage in prevention and treatment of overweight, obesity and their accompanying diseases.

1.2. WHAT INFLUENCES OUR WEIGHT, SHAPE AND HEALTH?

Weight and shape of the body is influenced by the volume and distribution of water, muscles, fat and other components of the body. The majority of body weight comprises water. However, water is a very unstable component, which is easily regulated by the organism itself or urination-regulating medication. It influences the overall body weight as well as the weight of individual organs. Once development is finished, it changes very little. The easiest to influence through exercise and protein diet is muscle mass. However, muscle mass causes relatively few health issues and the aesthetic ones trouble only bodybuilding enthusiasts and those who consider muscles a manifestation of masculinity. After all, musculature is a secondary sex marker and a marker of male reproductive hormones, affecting physical strength and fertility. Much more troubling for people is another component of the body – fat. In order to understand what fat causes (the good and the bad), what influences it and what we can and cannot do with it, you will need to endure some theory on physiology and pathology of obesity.

1.2.1. What Happens to the Food Inside Our Body?

What actually is metabolism and how does it influence the storing and expenditure of energy? Originally a Greek word, "metabolizmos" means "change." In our case it refers to the conversion of chemicals inside organisms. Life is a constant struggle with intake, conversion and loss of energy. In order to exist, living organisms require a constant intake of building materials and energy for their bodies and their correct functions. The source of both is nutrition. It contains primarily proteins, carbohydrates, and lipids, the conversion (metabolism) of which provides organisms with the building blocks and energy. All these components can be imagined as chains. In proteins, these consist of individual amino acids. Carbohydrates (polysaccharides) are formed from simple saccharides (monosaccharides) and lipids are chains of esters of fatty acids. Their composition is unique to each organism. During digestion, these chains are broken down to their components: proteins into amino acids, polysaccharides into monosaccharides, lipids into fatty acids and alcohol. During this process, energy is released. The elemental units are used as building blocks to produce materials natural to the organism. Amino acids are again formed into proteins required by the body, monosaccharides form polysaccharides and fatty acids form lipids. Besides that, carbohydrates can form from proteins (Schutz, 2011) and lipids from saccharides (Flatt, 1970, Schwarz, 2017). It happens at an increased rate during development, for example, but also in adulthood. The energy released during digestion is used in the process of digestion itself (to break down and reform molecules) but also to ensure other vital functions. When an organism takes in too much energy and nutrients, these accumulate in the organism as stores. From there, they can be released and used when necessary. The less energy you take in from food and the more of it you spend on basic functions, work and thermoregulation (dissipation of heat), the less of it is stored. It is stored in the form of lipids, polysaccharides (primarily the "animal starch" glycogen) and proteins. Synthesis of lipids requires the most energy and their breakdown releases the largest amounts of it. Therefore, lipids are the best energy stores. Excess lipids (fat) are stored in the cells of the so called white and brown adipose tissue primarily under the skin but also in the abdominal cavity and other parts of the body. Excess carbohydrates can accumulate in the liver not only as glycogen but also lipids, which cause lipidation (steatosis) of the liver (eSchwarz, 2017). The average fat stores of a human represent 10 to 12% of body weight, in obese people the percentage is higher (https://biopedia.sk/clovek/vyziva-a-metabolizmus, https://en.wikipedia.org/wiki/Lipid_metabolism). Women store 10 to 15% more fat than men and it accumulates in different parts of the body. Adipose tissue, in addition to being an energy store, functions also as surface thermal isolation. Lipids are an important component of cell walls. Adipose tissue acts as mechanical protection of the internal organs and produces hormones – adipokines, is a solvent of some vitamins and a source of water not only for camels but for people as well. Cells of the adipose tissue transform easily into other cells and can be utilized as stem cells (Haylett and Ferris, 2019, https://medaboutme.ru/obraz-zhizni/publikacii/stati/pohudenie/9_faktov_pro_zhir_na_nashem). The ratio of body fat and an optimal weight can be determined based on the Body Mass Index (BMI). BMI = weight (kg)/height (m)^2. World Health Organisation (WHO) provides the following BMI values to determine the degree of obesity (Mohamed et al., 2014):

<18.5 – malnutrition,
18.5-24.9 – normal weight,
25-29.9 – overweight,
30-34.9 – class I obesity,
35-39.9 – class II obesity,
40-44.9 – morbid obesity,
> 45 – superobesity.

It is easier to evaluate your weight and the related health risks based on the waist to hip ratio (WHR). Considered obese are men with WHR above 0.90 and women with WHR above 0.85. Men and women with WHR above 1.0 and above 0.80, respectively, are at increased risk of cardiovascular and other diseases connected to obesity (Mohamed et al., 2014).

A little more complicated is determination of fat stores based on biochemical analysis of blood. In blood serum, dietary fat and the lipids from adipose tissue are always present. Therefore, the levels of lipids and their metabolites (cholesterols and triacylglycerols) in blood can serve as a measurement for the total volume of fat in the body (https://en.wikipedia.org/wiki/Lipid_metabolism).

We hope that the results of your BMI, WHR and blood analysis cause you no wrinkles. And if they do – you are not alone; you belong to the 1.3 billion of our planet's inhabitants with overweight and obesity (Qussaada et al., 2019). It is important to be aware of this fact, understand its causes, and make an effort to limit its symptoms and negative consequences.

1.2.2. What Affects How Much Food We Eat and How We Use It?

Many of us envy those who can eat anything and gain no weight. And the other way around, women often complain they would gain weight even from eating air. Someone needs only a few spoonfuls of food for normal life while other people visit the fridge even at night. The cause of these differences lies in different effects of mechanisms regulating metabolic balance. I present some factors known to affect the body and its regulating systems. Now we know that the volume of fat depends on the balance between intake and expenditure of energy. Body guards this equilibrium through mechanisms of feedback, which stimulate appetite and energy preservation if the energy intake is too low and, on the other hand, cease the energy input (sensation of satiety), when its excessive. This regulation is performed by neuromediators in brain, neurohormones and hormones, nutrients themselves and gastrointestinal microbiota. These transfer the influence of outside factors (stress, temperature, biological rhythms, proprieties of food, etc.) to food intake and processing of nutrients and energy in our bodies (Mohamed et al., 2014, Nowak and Czkwianianc, 2016, Atawia et al., 2019, Barrea et al., 2019, Oussaada et al., 2019).

Such regulatory molecules are products of neurons – *neuromediators* serotonin and dopamine. Lack of calories decreases their levels in brain, which activates the centre of hunger. Conversely, food intake increases the levels of serotonin and dopamine, which triggers the feeling of happiness and euphoria. In addition to neuromediators, similarly involved in the regulation are *neurohormones*. Their (neuropeptide Y, orexin, encephalin, galanin, and others) production is stimulated by lack of food and consequently, they stimulate appetite. Full stomach suppresses the production of these hormones.

Further regulators of appetite are *hormones*, which are not produced in brains but in peripheral organs. Their production is affected by food intake and they, likely through the abovementioned neuromediators, act on the hunger centre in brain. For example, an empty stomach produces the hormone ghrelin, which upon entry into the brain activates the brain's hunger centre and incites the organism to eat. The hormone cortisol, produced by the adrenal glands under stress, also has a similar effect on appetite. Conversely, adipose tissue produces the hormone leptin. When there is enough fat, leptin suppresses the hunger centre in brain and activates the centre of happiness. At the same time, it activates the neurohormones in brain responsible for reproduction to produce offspring when conditions are favourable. Similar effects come from the hormones of pancreas (insulin, glucagon, pancreatic peptide, amylin, etc.) which are released under the influence of high levels of nutrients in blood. More than 20 hormones are produced in the intestines under the influence of food (cholecystokinin, peptide YY, xenin, etc.). All of them trigger the sensation of satiety, satisfaction, and prevent overeating. These hormones control lipid metabolism not just through the brain centres for food, hunger and happiness. They also regulate fat stores by their action on digestive processes, production of adipose cells, storing and burning of fat. Insensitivity of these hormones to presence of food can lead to disorders of the hormones-food feedback and consequently to metabolic disorders (obesity and likely also anorexia). Reproductive hormones regulate not only reproductive functions but also the sparing and expenditure of energy. Women have a more conservative metabolism, different volume and distribution of fat in the body and slower burning. Therefore, across all countries, obesity affects women more than men.

Metabolism-regulating neuromediators, neurohormones and peripheral hormones are influenced by *stress*. There is a direct link between the manifestation of obesity, stress (Tenk et al., 2018), lack of social success and unemployment (Blüher, 2019). Stress can stimulate eating and obesity directly through the brain centre as well as by stimulation of hypotalamo-hypophysal axis, which activates the release of the hormone cortisol. This hormone of the adrenal glands activates the hunger centre and suppresses the centres of satiety and happiness. In other words, it represses the mechanisms of food feedback. A person in distress overlooks that he or she has eaten enough already. Additionally, he or she consciously or subconsciously tries to neutralize frustration by activating the centre of happiness with food. Therefore, avoiding stress and tension during a meal is important in order for the feedback mechanisms to function correctly. First calm down in order to eat, not the other way around.

Food intake on the level of the brain and peripheries can be regulated not only by the neuromediators and hormones but by the *nutrients* themselves as well. For example, an increase in the glucose level in blood activates the abovementioned nervous and endocrinal mechanisms triggering the sensation of satiety and sparing of nutrients in stores.

Environmental *temperature* can have an even more important impact on fat stores than food intake, because it influences the burning of fat. Low temperatures demand from warm-blooded organisms the production of heat and burning of energy. Fat from brown adipose tissue is burned better than from white, which is more spared. Cold stimulates primarily the production of brown adipose tissue, even conversion (transformation) of white adipose tissue to brown (Giralt et al., 2013). Therefore, to treat obesity we need only a little – to find a method of converting white fat to brown and burning it without giving patients hypothermia. Recently, genes and molecules were discovered in mice that can achieve this even at normal temperatures (Dempersmier et al., 2015, Matesanz et al., 2018), but their application in humans is not yet known.

Activity of hunger centres is affected also by the *appearance, aroma and taste* of food, which impact the responsible neural centres through specific receptors. For example, people less sensitive to the taste of food, sugar and salt require more food to satisfy their receptors and have higher BMI. Therefore, avoid overuse of sugar and spices – over time, you will grow accustomed to them and will require more, which your body will reflect.

Storing and expenditure of energy depends considerably on *lifestyle*. Social status, education, sedentary lifestyle, sport, eating habits and vices have a strong impact on fat stores. For example, smokers have higher body weight than non-smokers (see further). In developing countries, women from higher social classes, who do not lack food, are larger than the poor ones. On the contrary, in developed countries obesity is characteristic for women with low level of education and income (Mohamed et al., 2014).

All physiological processes, including metabolism, have their own approximately 24-hour cycles called *circadian rhythms*. Every cell has a biological clock and they are synchronised by hypothalamus. However, rhythmic changes of the physiological functions must be compliant to the changes in the environment. Biological clock of an organism (including metabolism regulators) is set according to the circadian rhythms of two outside factors – lighting and food. Disruption of these circadian rhythms (for example by crossing of timezones, work at night, or irregular eating habits) can trigger metabolic disorders. Mice whose circadian rhythms of corticosteroids were artificially disrupted gained weight (Raghow, 2018). People working night shifts are at an increased risk of obesity and related diseases. Expenditure of energy to produce heat decreases over the course of the day. Therefore, after breakfast less energy is spared than after dinner (Paoli et al., 2019). Even a simple change of the eating schedule (while consuming the same food) can have a considerable impact on body weight. For example, it is not recommended to eat after 15-16 h (Oussaada et al., 2019, Paoli et al., 2019). Correctly set and maintained circadian rhythms of eating are essential for healthy metabolism.

All regulatory mechanisms and their functions are directed by *genes*. At present, scientists have identified at least 44 genes, the changes of which can facilitate hereditary or acquired obesity (Oussaada et al., 2019, Vettori et al., 2019). For example, obesity can be caused by insufficient activity of the p38α gene, which is responsible for the conversion of white adipose tissue to brown and its consequent burning in the form of heat (Matesanz et al., 2018). People with the risk variety of the FTO gene are 3-4 kg heavier and at 1.67 times the risk of obesity than people without the risk variety (Mohamed et al., 2014).

Naturally, the energy intake depends not only from the amount but the *calorie density* of food as well. Low-calorie diet improves metabolic parameters and reduces body weight (Zubrzycki et al., 2018). Calorie density of food depends on its composition. As described above, we gain the most energy from lipids, less from carbohydrates and the least from protein. People who consume more protein and less fat have lower BMI and WHR (Paoli et al., 2019). Therefore, mildly protein diets have their merit. On the other hand, proteins can be converted to fat and their increased consumption can lead to weight gain (Bray et al., 2012, Popp et al., 2019).

From the standpoint of weight gain, important is also the *digestibility* of lipids, carbohydrates and proteins. Digestion also requires energy, sometimes as much as a third of that taken in with food. Processing of easily digestible fatty acids, monosaccharides, and short-chain proteins requires less energy. Difficult to digest lipids, polysaccharides, and long-chain proteins require for their breakdown more energy, which would otherwise be spared in the fat stores. Therefore, aim for a correct ratio and form of these components in your diet. If you want to lose weight – eat more proteins and polysaccharides difficult to digest. If you need energy fast – eat fat and monosaccharides.

Last but not least, our metabolism depends not only on us but on foreign cells as well. In recent years, the irreplaceable role of *gastrointestinal microbiota* in storing energy and in obesity has been discovered. Gastrointestinal microbiota represents more cells and 150 times more genes than our own bodies comprise. They affect the nervous system and the manifestations of multiple nervous disorders (including depression, autism and anorexia). They help to digest substances such as fibre, which are difficult to digest or are indigestible by our own organism, from which they provide 5-10% of the necessary energy as well as a considerable amount of the molecules needed to synthesise lipids and saccharides. They increase nutrient absorption in the colon. In the breakdown of fibre by the bacteria of the large intestine, short-chain fatty acids are produced. These fatty acids are the source of energy for the gastrointestinal cells. Even more importantly, these acids activate oxidation of fatty acids in muscle mass, liver and brown adipose tissue and the dissipation of heat and consequently prevent storing of fat. Through their action on brain receptors, they suppress appetite. They support immunity and production of antibodies. These antibodies can bind to and inhibit hormones that trigger the sensation of hunger (Barrea et al.,

2019, Seitz et al., 2019). Loss of these bacteria causes disruptions in digestion and other vital functions. Many diseases are connected to the changes in gastrointestinal microbiota or in the absorption of bacterial products. On the other hand, manifestations of some metabolic diseases can be improved by the simple transplantation of gastrointestinal microbiota or their short-chain fatty acids from healthy individuals. Gastrointestinal bacteria are therefore not freeloaders and parasites, they are important partners in normalisation of metabolism, reduction of fat stores and obesity prevention. Therefore, support your gastrointestinal microbiota by consumption of fibre and unpasteurised dairy products containing beneficial lacto- and bifidobacteria. Do not panic when you or your children reach for something unsterilized. Instead, worry about the overuse of disinfection and antibiotics. These can massacre our small partners, who help maintain our metabolism and health.

The majority of validated data is related to factors regulating obesity. There are, however, indications that similar factors are responsible also for malnutrition caused by *anorexia nervosa*. People suffering from anorexia have altered brain centre activity, serotonin metabolism, levels of hormones responsible for food intake regulation (leptin, ghrelin, and other gastrointestinal hormones) and gastrointestinal microbiota (Seitz et al., 2019, Støving, 2019). Gastrointestinal microbiota can affect the levels of serotonin in the central nervous system. These are altered in patients with anorexia and return to normal levels with food intake (Seitz et al., 2019). These observations indicate that malnutrition due to *anorexia nervosa* can have the same regulators as normal nutrition. However, these correlations do not mean that these regulators are the cause of malnutrition rather than a reaction to it. Therefore, physiological mechanism of anorexia as well as the methods of its treatment are less known than in the case of obesity.

1.2.3. What Happens in Obesity, Why Is It Bad and How Can Be Avoid It?

Every disease is caused by too weak or excessively strong activity of regulators of physiological processes and an imbalance in their mutual relationships. Disorders of the lipid mechanism, including obesity, are no exception.

Adipose tissue is the largest store of energy in the body and also the largest endocrinal gland, which produces regulators – adipokines not only for itself but also for the entire mechanism. Obesity is a pathological hypertrophy (an unhealthy growth) of adipose tissue, which leads to many metabolic diseases (Mohamed et al., 2014, Atawia et al., 2019, Haider and Larose, 2019, Ghaben and Scherer, 2019). Obesity is caused by long-term imbalance between the intake and expenditure of energy, when excess energy is accumulated in the form of fat stores. Excessive fat stores weight down the organism and produce substances that cause of many diseases.

The volume of adipose tissue is increased in two ways: production of new adipose cells (adipocytes) or the already existing ones growing (hypertrophy). Of the two, multiplication of adipocytes is preferable. With multiplication of adipocytes, veins also develop, grow between the adipocytes in the adipose tissue and ensure healthy metabolism and production of adipokines. The role of adipokines (the regulators of adipose tissue) is to maintain the sensitivity of adipocytes to insulin and suppress manifestation of inflammatory processes. To adipokines belongs also the hormone leptin, which suppresses the centre of hunger (see previously). All these processes related to the multiplication and blood repletion of adipocytes promote metabolic balance.

Hypertrophy (increase in size) of adipocytes without the development of new veins leads to insufficient oxidation of the adipose cells, their fibrosis (thickening of the connective tissue), inflammation, and deterioration of adipocytes. The adipose tissue loses its function as an energy store and ceases to produce the necessary adipokines. This leads to decreased sensitivity to insulin and symptoms similar to diabetes. The levels of sugar and lipids in blood increase, they are stored in other organs (liver, muscles, and veins) and those then cease to function. This leads to a large spectrum of diseases – from cardiovascular diseases, disorders of immunity, to cancer. Insufficient adipocytes lead to a disruption in the feedback mechanisms by which the adipose tissue suppresses the hunger centre in brain. This leads to further overeating and increased obesity.

What the adipocytes choose – multiplication or increase in size – depends on multiple hormones (for example insulin, corticosteroids), growth and transcription factors and RNA interferences. For their detailed description, another book would be necessary. Understanding and application of these regulators, however, could help in management of adipose cells and obesity treatment. However, the selection can be influenced by us as well. For example, fasting reduces the growth of adipocytes, but the number of adipocytes remains unchanged.

In order to prevent overweight and obesity, it is possible to follow these simple rules for a healthy lifestyle:

- Be physically active every day (regular exercise, walking…).
- Aim for a diverse diet.
- Aim for regular defecation.
- Eat food rich in fibre.
- Gradually reduce food sizes. Chew carefully.
- Don't use gum. It stimulates the release of digestive juices and the feeling of hunger.
- Reduce animal fat and replace it with sources of "good fat" containing unsaturated fatty acids (plant-based oil, nuts)
- Avoid products made of white flour, white rice, salt and candy filled with simple carbohydrates and favour food containing polysaccharides and proteins (seeds, legumes, brown rice and wholegrain flour).
- Eat fresh fruit and vegetables every day.
- Avoid eating in the evening.
- Avoid antibiotics.
- Be content with your life.

Not everyone will relate to all these tips. Not all of them are possible to follow in everyday life. Nevertheless, their application can contribute to a healthy lifestyle and prevention of overweight and obesity.

1.2.4. Some Myths about Weight Loss

Among people, on the internet, and in literature, even the scientific, circulate many weight loss recipes. Some of them, however, should be taken with a grain of salt. Here are a few wide-spread beliefs about weight loss, which are not supported by the existing scientific knowledge.

1.2.4.1. If We Don't Eat Fat, We'll Be Healthy and Slim

Healthy – that will not happen without fats. As was already mentioned, body needs fat to store energy, for thermoregulation, mechanic protection for internal organs, as a building material for cells, as a source of hormones, a solvent for some substances, source of water, and likely also as a source of other cell types (Haylett and Ferris, 2019, https://medaboutme.ru/obraz-zhizni/publikacii/stati/pohudenie/9_faktov_
pro_zhir_na_nashem).

Slim – that is also questionable. Obesity can be facilitated not only by the consumption of fats, but proteins and carbohydrates as well. Lipids can be produced in metabolism of proteins (Schutz, 2011) and carbohydrates (Flatt, 1970; Schwartz, 2017). And if we consume large amounts of proteins and carbohydrates, these are burned instead of fat, which is then all stored instead of burned. Additionally, carbohydrates trigger production of insulin, which activates storing of fat (Bray, 2013). Therefore, fat stores can grow not only from fat intake, but from carbohydrates and proteins as well. For example, high protein intake from protein diets and during bodybuilding can lead to obesity instead of weight loss (Bray et al., 2012, Popp et al., 2019).

1.2.4.2. If I Skip Breakfast, I'll Lose Weight and Be Healthier

In some experiments, skipping breakfast aided in treatment of obesity (Geliebter et al., 2014), but other studies did not confirm this effect (Paoli et al., 2019). One reason can be that skipping breakfast disturbed the circadian rhythms of the metabolic process and reduced not only the intake but the expenditure of energy (as discussed earlier) as well. Some authors even state that skipping breakfast was linked to higher obesity rate, worse quality of nutrition (Ahadi et al., 2015; Monzani et al., 2019) and increased levels of fat and risk of cardiovascular diseases (Monzani et al., 2019, Paoli et al., 2019).

1.2.4.3. The More Often I Eat, the More Weight I Gain

What matters more is how much and what you eat. Number of daily meals evolves along with lifestyle (Paoli et al., 2019). Our ancestors – apes and hunters of the Stone Age – likely did not strictly divide meals into breakfast, lunch and dinner, but ate when food was available. The Ancient Romans ate usually only one meal at midday, and the medieval people – breakfast and lunch. It was only with the introduction of artificial lighting, which prolonged daily activities, that an evening meal became the social norm. Comparative studies of the prevalence of obesity showed better weight loss results for people eating 1-2 times a day and 5-6 times a day than those who ate 3 times a day (Paoli et al., 2019). Therefore, we can choose from two alternative models of eating. The first alternative is only one or two meals a day. This model can be better suited to busy people. The second model recommends 5 to 6 meals a day. Here, however, it is necessary to control the portion sizes of the individual meals in order to not exceed the optimum daily intake. Considering the physiology of digestion as well as the circadian rhythms, I lean towards the second model and recommend dividing the optimum daily energy intake into breakfast, lunch, dinner and a morning and afternoon snack.

1.2.4.4. Fasting Helps With Weight Loss

Not always. In fact, you can even gain weight during a fast (Paoli et al., 2019). The body resists the loss of energy stores by reducing energy expenditure (for heat production, physical activity, etc.) and increasing storing of fat after the fast. A religious fast (such as Lent or Rhamadan) does not always mean a decrease in the calorie intake, but only a change in the type of food consumed (meat replaced by fish, pasta, etc.) or a change from eating during the day to eating at night (which is not healthy). Despite that, it is widely practiced due to spiritual, cultural and religious reasons (Kralik et al., 2018). In the past, there were also economic reasons (fasting in spring, when there was little food). Roman emperors used to avoid food one day a month for health (Suetonius, 2010). Fasting can truly lead to reduction in weight, but only in combination with low-calorie diet (Zubrzycki et al., 2018). In some studies, fasting led to weight loss in all patients (Ganesan et al., 2018), in some, only in the obese ones but not the healthy ones. At the same time, the body weight returned to its original values at a rapid rate after fasting (Fernando et al., 2019).

1.2.4.5. With Healthy Lifestyle, Anyone Can Manage Healthy Weight Loss Or Gain

In theory, if I take in less energy and increase my expenditure of it, I will be losing weight. And the other way around. Therefore, the obesity epidemic is often connected to sedentary lifestyle. Long hours spent in front of television correlate with risk of obesity in both children and adults (Mohamed et al., 2014). For these reasons, limiting food intake and increasing physical activity are the most popular weight loss methods. In most cases it is even correct, but not always. First, hereditary obesity or thinness exist and they are not caused by incorrect eating habits but by damaged genes (polymorphism, mutations) regulating metabolism (Oussaada et al., 2019, Vettori et al., 2019). Second, a condition for weight loss is the combination of decreased energy intake and increased expenditure of it. To disrupt the equilibrium between these processes is very difficult not just psychologically but also physiologically. We have already described various interconnected feedback mechanisms, which guard the equilibrium between the intake and expenditure of energy and stabilize the energy stores of the organism. For example, the body reacts to decreased calorie intake by decreasing expenditure of energy and thus preserves the fat stores in an unchanged state (Paoli et al., 2019). Third, sport and exercise can increase energy expenditure to produce motion and heat. This expenditure, however, represents only a small percentage of the total energy output. The largest portion of energy expenditure is for basal metabolism (breathing, digestion, and thermoregulation). Basal metabolism is unique for each individual, hereditary, and difficult to influence (Oussaada et al., 2019). For example, the dissipation of heat is different between men and women. While women shake under a blanket at the height of summer, men wander around in shorts and t-shirts even in freezing temperatures. Therefore, men usually need for their muscles and thermoregulation much more food. Avoid long hours in front of TV or computer. But remember that your body will fight you and it has many objective reasons to be victorious in this struggle.

1.2.4.6. Physical Activity Burns Fat

Not always. Regular physical activity (sport, manual labour) activates at once the burning of fat, glycogen, and proteins. However, when a couch potato decides to start exercising, his body will first burn glycogen, then proteins and finally fat. Therefore, he'll need more time and effort to burn fat than a person who is regularly physically active. If he burns any fat at all (Haylett and Ferris, 2019, https://medaboutme.ru/obraz-zhizni/publikacii/ stati/pohudenie/9_faktov_pro_zhir_na_nashem).

1.2.4.7. Smoking is Slimming

This myth is based on the fact that people who stop smoking often gain weight. That is, however, a result of an overall improvement in health and that these people exchange one vice for another (instead of a cigarette, they reach for candy). In reality, smokers (regardless of the number of cigarettes smoked daily) gain approximately 4.4 (men) and 5.0 (women) kg more over 10 years than non-smokers (Mohamed et al., 2014).

I hope this information will spare you false hope and unnecessary disappointment when engaging in activities that might not bring desired results. On the other hand, I believe this knowledge can help you define and manage a healthy lifestyle. And individual obesity treatment should be consulted with experts – medical doctors.

Chapter 2

SELECTED PLANTS AND THEIR MOLECULES, WHICH CAN IMPACT FAT STORES

2.1. INTRODUCTION: HOW CAN PLANTS HELP IN WEIGHT LOSS?

Analysis of scientific literature shows that storing of fat and excess weight can be efficiently repressed by products which decrease appetite or reduce the levels of lipids in blood and internal organs. Obesity can be counteracted, in addition to physical activity and healthy lifestyle, by consumption of plant products with the following characteristics: (Björck and Elmståhl, 2003, Pittler and Ernst, 2004; Cherniack, 2008; Hasani-Ranjbar et al., 2012: Smith et al., 2012; Fardet and Chardigny, 2013; Yasueda et al., 2013; Gamboa-Gómez et al., 2015, Ríos-Hoyo and Gutiérrez-Salmeán, 2016; Lu et al., 2018):

- plants, which contain few easily digestible molecules (monosaccharides) and a lot ones difficult to digest (polysaccharides, fibre), which trigger the sensation of satiety,

- plant molecules which repress production, proliferation and differentiation of adipose cells
- plant molecules which decrease the activity of enzymes responsible for the production of lipids and high levels of triacylglycerols in blood
- plant molecules which increase the activity of enzymes responsible for conversion of white adipose tissue into brown, which increases the burning of fat, its oxidation and conversion of stored fat into heat
- plant molecules which repress the absorption of lipids
- plant molecules which suppress the activity of hunger centres in brain
- plant preparations which activate the centres of sweetness on tongue and then repress the feeling of hunger without considerable calorie intake
- plant molecules which slow down bowel discharge and create a sensation of satiety
- plant substances (saccharides, fibre) – prebiotics which support the gastrointestinal microbiota, which produce short-chain fatty acids and trigger the feeling of a full stomach

The following chapters are dedicated to a critical analysis of individual plants, their components and combinations which can influence these metabolic processes and could be applicable in weight reduction and improved health of humans.

2.2. APPLE CIDER VINEGAR

2.2.1. Introduction: Provenance and Properties

Apple cider vinegar is made of apples (*Malus domestica*), which have undergone bacterial fermentation – a process in which sugar is first converted to alcohol (for example in production of cider) and that is then fermented to acetic acid. Besides apple cider vinegar, the product of apple fermentations contains also other biologically active components – gallic acid, catechin Y, epicatechins and chlorogenic acid, caffeic acid, p-Coumaric acid, ferulic acid, citric acid, and folic acid. It also contains phosphor, calcium, copper, sodium, potassium, vitamins A, B1, B2, B6, C, E, pectin, mineral salts, amino acids and flavonoids with antioxidant effect (Budak et al., 2014, https://www.zdravieastyl.sk/potraviny-a-vyziva/193-sila-jablcneho-octu).

2.2.2. Positive Effects on Human Health

Apple cider vinegar has antioxidant, antimicrobial, anti-tumour, antidiabetic and other effects beneficial to health (Budak et al., 2014). It lowers blood pressure and treats hypertonia (Kondo et al., 2001). Thanks to its antioxidant effect, it prevents oxidative stress and the related damage to internal organs and diseases linked to oxidative stress (Nazıroğlu et al., 2014). It can improve the condition of gastrointestinal tract and digestion (Suiryanrayna and Ramana, 2015, http://dni.skwww.plusden.sk/zena/chudnutie/dieta-tento-tyzden/jablcny-ocot-naozaj-roztopi-tuk-potvrdili-aj-vedci.html). It reduces the concentration of glucose and insulin in blood, especially after meals high in carbohydrates (Liljeberg and Björck, 1998, Fushimi et al., 2005, Johnston and Buller, 2005, Sakakibara et al., 2006, Petsiou et al., 2014, Russell et al., 2016, Shishehbor et al., 2017, Siddiqui et al., 2018). Therefore, it is considered a prospective natural treatment against diabetes (Russell et al., 2016, Yamashita et al., 2016, Siddiqui, 2018).

2.2.3. Positive Effects on Weight Reduction

It can serve as an efficient tool in weight loss (Johnston, 2005, Kondo et al., 2009, Yamashita, 2016) as it reduces weight through several mechanisms:

- It suppresses the centre of hunger in the central nervous system (Frost et al., 2014) and reduces appetite (Johnston, 2005, Darzi et al., 2014),
- It reduces the level of saccharides and lipids in blood, which act on the centre of hunger (see above)
- It is assumed that it could slow faecal output after a meal and therefore extend the sensation of satiety (Liljeberg and Björck, 1998),
- It activates genes and the enzyme AMPK (activated protein kinase), which stimulates burning of fat (Sakakibara et al., 2006, Yamashita, 2016),
- It reduces production and accumulation of lipids in the body and liver (Johnston, 2005 Darzi et al., 2014, Yamashita, 2016, Yamashita et al., 2016)

In both the obese (Kondo et al., 2009) and healthy (Darzi et al., 2014) people, consumption of apple cider vinegar reduced body weight, volume of fat and level of triacylglycerols in blood. Nazıroğlu et al., (2014), on the other hand, determined in mice that this vinegar, due to its antioxidant effect, prevented oxidation of lipids in internal organs.

In addition to acetic acid, involved in weight reduction might be also another component of apple cider vinegar – vitamin C. People with higher concentration of vitamin C oxidate 30% more lipids during physical activity than people with lower concentration (Johnston, 2005).

2.2.4. Possible Adverse Side-Effects

Excessive doses of acetic acid can cause adverse side-effects such as stomach irritation, heartburn, and irritated throat (Hill et al., 2005, (https://sk.thefreespiritedwoman.com/1888-5-side-effects-of-apple-cider-vinegar-nobody-told-you-about), tooth decay (Gambon et al., 2012, https://sk.thefreespiritedwoman.com/1888-5-side-effects-of-apple-cider-vinegar-nobody-told-you-about), nausea (Darzi et al., 2014) and increased risk of diabetes (https://sk.thefreespiritedwoman.com/1888-5-side-effects-of-apple-cider-vinegar-nobody-told-you-about). Hypocalcaemia can cause osteoporosis (reduced bone density, bone thinning) as well as constipation, muscle weakness, abnormal heart rhythm and exhaustion (https://sk.simpleaslife.com/20805-side-effects-of-apple-cider-vinegar-tablets.html).

Acetic acid can alter the effects of some medication – insulin, digoxin, diuretics, furosemide, torsemide and bumetanide, there it is not recommended to combine them. (https://sk.simpleaslife.com/20805-side-effects-of-apple-cider-vinegar-tablets.html).

2.2.5. General Evaluation and Recommendations

Previous research carried out on laboratory animals and livestock as well as humans (both healthy and suffering from obesity and diabetes) conclusively validated the application of apple cider vinegar and its molecules had positive effects on numerous physiological processes and health. In particular, reduction of fat stores and body weight. Application of apple cider vinegar at a dose of 45 ml a day should be beneficial for normalisation of fat stores and body weight without adverse side-effects.

2.3. CAROB (*CERATONIA SILIQUA* L.).

2.3.1. Introduction: Provenance and Properties

Carob (*Ceratonia siliqua* L.) is an evergreen tree of medium height from the *Fabaceae* (pea) family. The precise origin of the plant is not known, but it has been grown in Ancient Egypt as early as 2000 BC. It probably came from the region of Middle East. From there, carob spread into the Mediterranean regions and nowadays it is grown in all tropical areas. The Spanish introduced carob to Mexico and South America, the British to South Africa, India and Australia. Its name (carob) is of Arabic origin. The female flowers will develop into 12-30 cm long brown pods with sweet pulp, which are called *Ceratoniae fructus, Siliqua dulcis*, locust bean or St John's-bread. According to a legend, they were St. John's sustenance in desert. Seeds of carob were in the past used as weights on scales to weight gems or gold. The unit name carat (0.2 g) is therefore derived from the word carob.

Carob beans are high (87.54% of dry matter) in saccharides, including difficult to digest polysaccharides galactomannans ("soluble fibre"), in proteins, A and B vitamins, microelements (K, P, Ca, Mg, Fe, Mn, Zn, Cu), insoluble fibre, polyphenols with antioxidant effect (catechins, quercin, gallic acid), carotenoids, and contain essentially no lipids (Khatib et al., 2010, Lakkab et al., 2010, Dionísio and Grenha, 2012, Karim and Azlan, 2012, Rtibi et al., 2017, Rico et al., 2019). Due to the high saccharide content and sweet taste and aroma, they are often used in production of chocolate, candy, baked goods, beverages, in processing of meat, milk, fruit and vegetables, cosmetic products, and the fruit brandy rakia (Croatian "rakija od rogača"). Isolated from the pods containing galactomannan is locust bean gum, which is a permitted natural food additive under the number E-410 https://sk.wikipedia.org/wiki/Rohovn%C3%ADk_oby%C4%8Dajn%C3%BD, https://hl.rs/suche-zlato-mediteranu/, http://www.minevita.sk/sk/oznamy/clanky/rohovnik-obycajny.html) .

2.3.2. Positive Effects on Human Health

Carob is a healthier alternative to cocoa not only thanks to its colour but also taste. Although it cannot entirely replace the typical chocolate taste, it is suitable for use in ice cream, baking, cooking, etc. In comparison to cocoa, it is three times richer in calcium, one third lower in calories and contains seven times less fat and almost no theobromine, methylxanthine damaging to health and allergenic molecules. Its consumption therefore does not cause an increased pulse rate, sleep disorders and hyperactivity. Therefore, it is recommended for children, people suffering from insomnia, allergies to cocoa and chocolate, celiac disease and osteoporosis, and those who require high calcium intake (https://www.fragrantica.com/notes/Carob-tree-

430.html). Carob chocolate is suitable not only for people suffering from milk or cocoa allergies, but also for everyone who would like to pleasantly enrich their diet (https://hl.rs/suche-zlato-mediteranu/).

Thanks to its content of insoluble as well as soluble fibre (galactomannans), carob stops diarrhoea, reduces bad LDL cholesterol in blood of animals (El Rabey et al., 2017) and humans (Zunft et al., 2003, Ruiz-Roso et al., 2010), by which it prevents many other civilisation diseases. It also helps in digestion and defecation, detoxication and normalisation of gastrointestinal microbiota. Carob polyphenols are similar to molecules contained in tea (but it does not contain caffeine) and have also similar antioxidant activity. They can inhibit multiplication of cancer cells and have antidepressant as well as sedating effects (Karim and Azlan, 2012, Rtibi et al., 2017, Jamous et al., 2018, Lakkab et al., 2018). Additionally, carob reduced markers of hypertension and inflammations in animals (Martínez-Villaluenga et al., 2018, Rico et al., 2019).

2.3.3. Positive Effects on Weight Reduction

Thanks to low fat and calorie content, carob can be considered healthy and light food, which has the potential to prevent weight gain. Carob has naturally sweet taste, therefore the food it is added to requires less sweetening. Additionally, carob contains also fibre and polyphenols, which in previous experiments prevented obesity (see descriptions of other molecules countering obesity) and reduced LDL cholesterol's concentration in blood of animals (El Rabey et al., 2017) and people (Zunft et al., 2003). They also reduced storing of fat in cultured adipocytes (Martínez-Villaluenga et al., 2018, Rico et al., 2019). These observations indicate that carob can be applied to reduce fat stores in the body and treat obesity. Unfortunately, the only clinical study carried out up to date has not validated a statistically significant effect of carob meal consumption on cholesterol levels (total and LDL) in blood of obese patients and in certain cases the levels were actually increased (Martínez-Rodríguez et al., 2013). The ability of carob molecules to repress enzymes which break down lipids was validated also by *in vitro* experiments (Jamous et al., 2018). It cannot be excluded that decreased cholesterol under carob's influence in some experiments on animals was caused by inhibition of its solution and not by reduction of the volume of fat – its source.

Therefore, the results of the studies carried out so far are contradictory and have not validated the ability of carob molecules to positively affect fat stores and obesity in humans.

2.3.4. Possible Adverse Side-Effects

Literature reports no serious adverse side-effects of carob on health of animals and humans.

2.3.5. General Evaluation and Recommendations

Carob can be considered healthy, light and health-beneficial food. It can be unavoidable in the case of people for whom cocoa, chocolate or caffeine intake is undesirable. Studies of carob consumption on reduction of fat stores and body weight are insufficient and the results collected from them did not validate a positive effect on lipid metabolism and weight loss in humans.

2.4. COFFEE
(*COFFEA ARABICA* AND *COFFEA CANEPHORA*)

2.4.1. Introduction: Provenance and Properties

Coffee plant (*Coffea spp.*) is a short tree or a bush native to Africa, the fruits of which are red coffee "cherries." The best-known molecule in this fruit is alkaloid methylxanthine caffeine (1,3,7 trimetylxantin) – a toxin, which protects the plant from herbivores. In addition to caffeine, coffee fruit contains alkaloid trigonelline, polyphenol chlorogenic acid, ferulic acid, diterpenes cafestrol and kahweol, melanoidins and coffee lipids (Ludwig et al., 2014, Islam et al., 2018, Stefanello et al., 2018).

2.4.2. Positive Effects on Human Health

Clinical studies demonstrated that the ability of coffee to reduce blood sugar is not dependent on caffeine but on its other components (Tunnicliffe and Shearer, 2008). This effect probably comes from chlorogenic acid. Chlorogenic acid has antioxidant and anti-inflammatory effects, it can affect metabolism of glucose and lipids. Thanks to its antioxidant, anti-inflammatory and metabolic effects, coffee and its molecule chlorogenic acid have a preventive and therapeutic influence against diabetes, cardiovascular diseases, tumours, inflammation, lipidation of liver and Parkinson disease (Ludvig et al., 2014, Tajik et al., 2017, Islam et al., 2018, Perumpail et al., 2018). Their consumption can be recommended to healthy people and people with high cholesterol and blood sugar, with hypertension, and to prevent metabolic syndrome (Sarriá et al., 2018, Xie et al., 2018) and diabetes (Tunnicliffe and Shearer, 2008). Anti-diabetic effects were determined not only in chlorogenic acid but in other acid components of coffee – caffeine and ferulic acid – as well (Islam et al., 2018).

Large-scale studies showed a correlation between the habit of drinking coffee and reduced mortality linked to cardiovascular diseases, reduced risk of heart attacks, diabetes and some types of tumours. Contrary to popular belief, drinking coffee was not linked to increased occurrence of cardiac arrhythmias – in fact, not even a negative correlation of these phenomena was determined (Bhatti et al., 2013). Thanks to the ability of coffee's antioxidants to bind free radicals (Yashin et al., 2013) and reduce diseases and mortality, coffee earned the title "longevity beverage" (Bhatti et al., 2013).

2.4.3. Positive Effects on Weight Reduction

Coffee reduces storing of fat in the body by several mechanisms:

- It inhibits multiplication of adipocytes
- It influences transcription factors and other proteins involved in production of lipids in these cells
- Through action on gastrointestinal microbiota, which can also affect obesity (Pan et al., 2016).

Thanks to these effects, coffee can reduce fat stores in obese animals and humans (Hasani-Ranjbar et al., 2009, Onakpoya et al., 2011, Pan et al., 2016, Ríos-Hoyo and Gutiérrez-Salmeán, 2018, Tabrizi et al., 2019) and reduce body weight of humans (Hasani-Ranjbar et al., 2009, Onakpoya et al., 2011, Pan et al., 2016, Tabrizi et al., 2019). A study of Sarriá et al. (2018) determined a positive effect of green and roasted coffee on metabolic indexes but not on body weight of patients.

2.4.4. Possible Adverse Side-Effects

Caffeine in large doses can cause anxiety, insomnia, loss of calcium from the body and consequent increased risk of fractures, especially in people with osteoporosis (Bhatti et al., 2013). Possible negative effects of caffeine on brain development and development of reproductive organs in embryos and children have not been excluded (Islam et al., 2018). There are indications that caffeine and coffee can damage sperm and prolong pregnancy (Ricci et al., 2017). Cafestrol and kahweol can increase levels of blood cholesterol (de Roos et al., 1999). Despite these factors, large-scale studies found no statistically significant effect of coffee and caffeine consumption on the occurrence of health complications in adults, pregnant women, adolescents and children (Doepker et al., 2018) and conversely, they determined positive effect on health and longevity (see above).

2.4.5. General Evaluation and Recommendations

The results of our analysis of scientific literature validate coffee extract's application for weight loss and treatment of some metabolic disorders (diabetes, obesity, etc.). Coffee has a number of other positive physiological effects on health and longevity. Adverse side-effects of coffee are not serious and they manifest only when consumption is excessive. This knowledge allows to recommend coffee extract as an ingredient in a beverage intended for weight loss.

At present, the market offers numerous kinds of coffee. Naturally, a question arises as to which are the most efficient for weight reduction and at what dose.

2.4.5.1. Is Green Coffee Better For Weight Loss Then Roasted?

Marketers of green coffee claim that "Green coffee... contains more antioxidants and acids. Roasting destroys a large amount" (https://www.rexter.cz/rubriky/zajimavosti/ucinky-piti-kavy-na-nase-zdravi_165.html). "Because the beans were not subjected to high temperatures, they did not lose some beneficial components, which degrade in roasting" (https://zaujimavosti.net/ blog/je-zelena-kava-podvod-alebo-naozaj-funguje-jej-efekt-pri-spalovani-tukov). These claims are not compliant with scientific knowledge. During roasting of green coffee, so called Mallard Reaction metabolizes chlorogenic acid to antioxidant melanoid, which is responsible for the biological activity of this acid (Tunnicliffe and Shearer, 2008, Dybkowska et al., 2017). Green coffee contains fewer antioxidants and polyphenols than roasted (Odžaković et al., 2016). This means that roasting increases rather than reduces the metabolic effecs of coffee.

2.4.5.2. Is Decaffeinated Coffee Better For Weight Loss?

Decaffeination decreases the antioxidant activity of coffee (Yashin et al., 2013). Tunnicliffe and Shearer (2008) proved that positive effects of coffee are not dependent on caffeine at all but instead on other components.

Therefore, in relation to weight loss the presence or absence of caffeine in your coffee makes no difference.

2.4.5.3. How Much Coffee to Drink for Weight Reduction?

Popular websites recommend to patients: "Optimum coffee intake is up to 300 mg, which represents 3-6 cups of coffee a day. Caffeine content in 1 coffee, however, depends also on the type of consumed coffee. For example, one cup of instant coffee contains 50-60 mg of caffeine, drip coffee 80-100 mg and presso 90-150 mg" (https://www.slovenskypacient.sk/kava-a-zdravie-desat-prinosov-kavy/). Another website recommends "Four cups of coffee, which represent approximately 400 mg caffeine a day, provide maximum effect" (https://www.mayoclinic.org/healthy-lifestyle/nutrition-and-healthy-eating/in-depth/caffeine/art-20045678, http://www.pluska.sk/izdravie/archiv/zdravie/prevratne-zistenia-kave-kolko-salok-denne-je-zdravych.html). These recommendations are compliant with the scientific data. One strong cup of coffee contains 60 mg of pure chlorogenic acid. This dose has essentially no effect on absorption of chlorogenic acid into the body (Williamson et al., 2011). At this dose, any physiological effect is unlikely. Metabolic effect is achieved at daily intake of minimum 510.6 mg of chlorogenic acid and 121.2 mg of caffeine (Sarriá et al., 2018), which represents approximately 3 cups. In Canada, considered a safe dose for adults are 400 mg of caffeine and 10 g for one-time dose (Doepker et al., 2018). Drinking 5 cups of coffee a day had only positive effects on health (Carlström et al., 2018). Therefore, a dose of 2.5-5 cups of coffee containing 400 mg of caffeine a day can be considered a metabolically efficient as well as safe dose. For those who cannot possibly manage that many coffees a day, coffee can be replaced by an adequate amount of chlorogenic acid and caffeine.

This evidence speaks in favour of roasted coffee extract with caffeine at a dose of 2.5-5 cups of coffee a day to be used for weight reduction.

2.5. CINNAMON

2.5.1. Introduction: Provenance and Properties

The cinnamon family (*Laureaciae*) comprises more than 300 species of evergreen trees or bushes growing in America, Asia, Oceania and Australia (https://www.revolvy.com/page/Cinnamomum). In culinary arts and medicine, the most commonly used are 2 species - *Cinnamomum zeylanicum* (=*Cinnamomum verum*) and *Cinnamon cassia* (=*Cinnamomum aromaticum*). They contain biologically active molecules cinnamaldehydes, cinnamic acid, cinnamate, many other polyphenols, antioxidants, manganese, iron, calcium and fibre. Cinnamon molecules have antioxidant, anti-inflammation, anti-diabetic, antimicrobial and anticarcinogenic effects. There are data on their ability to prevent and treat cancer, inflammation, cardiovascular and neurological diseases of the Parkinson and Alzheimer type (Rao and Gan, 2014, Hariri and Ghiasvand, 2016, Santos and da Silva, 2018).

2.5.2. Positive Effects on Human Health

Cinnamon's molecules cinnamaldehyde and cinnamic acid have medicinal effects. As antioxidants, they bind free radicals. They reduce levels of glucose and cholesterol in blood, soothe pain, inflammation, stomach ulcers, suppress growth of bacteria and fungi. Through a number of signalling molecules (Dorri et al., 2018, Kawatra and Rajagopalan, 2015, Hosni et al., 2017, Hajimonfarednejad et al., 2018, Van Hul et al., 2018), they increase the body's resistance to the effect of natural and chemical poisons in liver, kidneys, blood, brain, heart, spleen, reproductive system.

From the standpoint of improving carbohydrate metabolism and body weight reduction, important are the data on cinnamon's ability to reduce production and absorption of glucose in intestines, increase glucose metabolism and glycogen synthesis, stimulate insulin production, activate insulin receptors and reduce levels of glucose and cholesterol in blood

(Ranasinghe et al., 2012). Therefore, it is considered a prospective natural treatment against diabetes (Medagama, 2015, Santos et al., 2018). On the other hand, other publications did not validate cinnamon's ability to alter glucose metabolism (Whitfield et al., 2016) or levels of insulin and inflammation markers in blood (Liu et al., 2015).

2.5.3. Positive Effects on Weight Reduction

Cinnamon can reduce fat stores in the body through several pathways:

- reduces serotonin production in brain, which can suppress the activity of the hunger centre (Bano et al., 2014)
- suppresses production of "hunger hormone" ghrelin and therefore reduces appetite (Camacho et al., 2015)
- regulates enzymes and molecules responsible for lipid production and decreases their level in blood and accumulation in cells (Liu et al., 2018)
- activates genes responsible for oxidation (burning) of fat (Camacho et al., 2015, Lu et al., 2018). Released energy is dissipated in the form of heat (Abeysekera et al., 2017, Jiang et al., 2017)
- triggers death of adipose cells (Lu et al., 2018),

Probably due to these processes, consumption of cinnamon reduces appetite (Hochkogler et al., 2018) and facilitates weight loss (Uragoda, 1984, Whitfield et al., 2016, Liu et al., 2018, https://www.rd.com/health/diet-weight-loss/cinnamon-weight-loss/). On the other hand, in some studies, cinnamon did not affect the ratio of LDL and HDL cholesterol (Maierean et al., 2017) and levels of lipids in blood (Liu et al., 2015). In some experiments, cinnamon treatment had no effect on body weight of people with obesity, but ratio of lipids and other components in the body was altered (Liu et al., 2015). Conversely, Markey et al. (2011) did not determine any influence of cinnamon on oxidation, metabolism and appetite in humans.

It needs to be mentioned that consumption of cinnamon by female rats triggered metabolic disorders and obesity in their offspring (Neto et al., 2019). This could imply possible danger for pregnant women consuming cinnamon.

2.5.4. Possible Adverse Side-Effects

Aldehyde cinnamic can irritate. Long-term consumption of large doses of cinnamon can lead to asthma, gastrointestinal tract dysfunctions and allergic reactions (Uragoda, 1984, Isaac-Renton et al., 2015, Hajimonfarednejad et al., 2018). Worse consequence can be caused by the presence of coumarin in cinnamon, because it is toxic to liver and kidneys. Even short-term consumption of müssli with cinnamon can trigger dangerous accumulation of coumarin in the body (Fotland et al., 2012). *Cinnamomum zeylanicum* contains significantly less coumarin than *Cinnamomum cassia* (Medagama, 2015). We already mentioned the ability of cinnamon to trigger metabolic disorders in offspring (Neto et al., 2019).

2.5.5. General Evaluation and Recommendations

Positive effect of cinnamon and its components for weight loss is validated in the majority of performed studies. Adverse side-effects can by caused only by a component of cinnamon – coumarin. Therefore, the use of cinnamon in weight loss can be justified.

A problem with cinnamon consumption at large doses can be the toxic effect of the contained coumarin. *Cinnamomum cassia* contains significantly more coumarin toxin than *Cinnamomum zeylanicum*. Therefore, I recommend the use of the less toxic *Cinnamomum zeylanicum*.

2.6. CHIA (*SALVIA HISPANICA* L.)

2.6.1. Introduction: Provenance and Properties

Chia (*Salvia hispanica* L.) and a lesser-known related species "golden chia" (*Salvia columbariae*) belong to the *Lamiaceace* family. In Central America, they were cultivated already by the Aztecs as edible and medicinal plants. Their economic importance was similar to that of cereals and maize. Currently, they are grown in South America, the USA and Australia (Valdivia-López and Tecante, 2015, https://en.wikipedia.org/wiki/Chia_seed). Their dry seeds are rich in vitamins, minerals, soluble fibre, proteins and fat, fatty acids, primarily unsaturated, among which notable is linoleic acid (an essential acid our bodies cannot synthetize themselves) and omega-3 and omega-6 fatty acids beneficial to health (Marcinek and Krejpcio, 2017, Parker et al., 2018, https://ndb.nal.usda.gov/ndb/search/list?qlookup=12006&format=Full).

2.6.2. Positive Effects on Human Health

Consumption of chia seeds and their lipids had a similar positive effect on health (Parker et al., 2018). Documented are prophylactic effects of chia seeds and their molecules on hypertension, cardiovascular diseases, cancer and diabetes (Marcinek and Krejpcio, 2017). They can reduce hypertension (de Souza Ferreira et al, 2015) and suppress manifestations of inflammation (Vuksan et al., 2017). There are data about their capability to reduce blood sugar (Parker et al., 2018), although this effect is not confirmed by all studies (Tavares Toscano et al., 2014). They suppress itching of skin. They increase the performance and stamina of athletes (Parker et al., 2018).

2.6.3. Positive Effects on Weight Reduction

Chia seeds are able to absorb a large volume of water and produce gel. Therefore, we can assume they can fill the gastrointestinal tract and trigger the feeling of satiety without calorie intake. At the same time, the high content of fatty acids in chia seeds (see above) suggests their positive effect on metabolism of lipids and weight loss. So far, these presumptions have not been sufficiently validated by science experiments. Some tests demonstrated the ability of chia to reduce cholesterol (Tavares Toscano et al., 2014) and body weight of people with obesity (Tavares Toscano et al., 2014, Vuksan et al., 2017, Parker et al., 2018). Similar effect was achieved also by treatment with chia in combination with other plant molecules in obese patients (Balliett et al., 2013). Some of these studies were not statistically significant (de Souza Ferreira et al., 2015). In other experiments, the consumption of chia oil or seeds reduced the levels of lipids in blood (Oliveira-de-Lira et al., 2018) but had no influence on body weight (Nieman et al., 2009, Ulbricht et al., 2009, Oliveira-de-Lira et al., 2018). Therefore, the effect of chia on weight loss cannot yet be considered conclusively proven.

2.6.4. Possible Adverse Side-Effects

As of yet, no undesirable adverse side-effects of chia were determined even in combination with other medication (Ulbricht et al., 2009).

2.6.5. General Evaluation and Recommendations

It cannot be excluded that an introduction of chia into diet can have a positive effect on prevention of some diseases and health complications including metabolic dysfunctions. No negative effects are presumed. On the other hand, the ability of chia to affect human metabolism has not been sufficiently studied and its effect on body weight remains questionable. Therefore, it is premature to assume it can help treat body weight issues.

2.7. Chicory (*Cichorium intybus* L.) and Its Molecule Inulin

2.7.1. Introduction: Provenance and Properties

Common chicory (*Cichorium intybus L.*) (known also under the common names blue daisy, blue sailors, blue weed, coffee weed, cornflower, horseweed, ragged sailors, succory, wild bachelor's buttons, wild endive, and witloof) belongs to the family *Cichoriaceae*, or according to other sources to the family *Asteraceae*. From its native Mediterranean region, this undemanding weed spread into the entire Europe and Asia. Chicory is a perennial herb, which can grow up to 1 m tall. It has been known already in Ancient Egypt, where it was considered magical and able to bring beauty and success. Chicory grows freely in the wild, but it is grown also in gardens as a root crop, honey plant, herb and food with added value. At present, chicory in Slovakia is grown for its root, which is used in the food industry, for example to produce decaffeinated coffee.

In addition to the commonly-known chicory with light blue flowers, grown are also the following varieties (Street et al., 2013, https://zdravina.sk/cakanka-obycajna/):

- White – which is referred to also as "white gold" and is popular especially in Belgium, the Netherlands and England. It contains inulin (fibre I describe later) and molecules stimulating blood production and circulation. Of vitamins, present in the plant are B vitamins, C vitamin, of the minerals potassium, phosphor and calcium. It is used in salads but is suitable also for baking.

- Red – comes from Italy. It contains primarily vitamin B1, beta-carotene, folic acid, iron, phosphor, potassium, zinc and fibre. It is suitable for salad preparation.
- Lettuce – it is similar to lettuce in appearance, which is where its name comes from. It contains C vitamin, stimulates appetite, and influences activity of intestines. It is suitable for salads, cooking and braising.
- Loose-Leaf chicory with fine leaves, which are used like lettuce.

Chicory root comprises up to 49% inulin, 0.1% glycoside intybin, tannins, choline, arginine, resin, mucus, minerals. The main containing substances are in its latex. These are bitter terpene substances, triterpene derivates, gum, etc. In leaves: coumarin glycoside cichorine, also levulose, inulin, choline, arginine, cichoric acid. These molecules stimulate specific characteristics of baked chicory's taste and aroma as well as its effects on health (Street et al., 2013, https://www.nazdravie.sk/cakanka-obycajna/, https://zdravina.sk/cakanka-obycajna/).

From the standpoint of health, the most important is high inulin content in roots, which in turns into caramel during baking. Inulin is a storage polysaccharide of inulin-containing crops. Besides chicory, it is found in Jerusalem artichoke, dahlia, onion, garlic, asparagus, leek, banana, agave, artichokes, and another 36 000 species (Shoaib et al., 2016, Korczak and Slavin 2018, Vollmannová et al., 2018). It is produced primarily by polymerisation fructose units. It is naturally mildly sweet. While it is soluble in water, it is not digestible in stomach and small intestine. The gastrointestinal microbiota breaks it down partially. Therefore, it is considered "soluble fibre" and a prebiotic, which provides sustenance for lactobacteria and bifidobacteria and enables their multiplication in colon (Roberfroid, 1999, Flamm et al., 2001, Shoaib et al., 2016, Wilson and Whelan K, 2017).

Through enzymatic hydrolyse of inulin, fructoolygosaccharides, used as a strong artificial sweetener, are produced. These are hydrolysed by enzymes of the gastrointestinal system (Flamm et al., 2001, Mensink et al., 2015, Vollmannová et al., 2018).

2.7.2. Positive Effects on Human Health

In traditional as well as official medicine, chicory and its molecules are used to treat the following diseases (Roberfroid, 1999, https://www.zdravieastyl.sk/prirodna-medicina/23-cakanka-obycajna, https://zdravoteka.sk/byliny/cakanka-obycajna/, https://www.zdravieastyl.sk/prirodna-medicina/23-cakanka-obycajna):

- Kidney stones
- Urinary tract inflammation
- Varicose ulcer
- Respiratory diseases
- Diseases of gastrointestinal tract
- Diseases of retina
- Kidney diseases
- Diseases of galbladder and bile ducts
- Liver diseases
- Infectious skin disorders
- Hair disorders
- Diseases of conjunctiva
- Eczema
- Irritations of the eye
- Swollen joints
- Constipation
- Blisters
- Ulcers
- Rashes

Inulin alters activity of central nervous system (CNS) (Anastasovska et al., 2012) and gastrointestinal microbiota's composition (Anastasovska et al., 2012, Reimer et al., 2017). It is presumed that CNS as well as gastrointestinal bacteria can transfer inulin action on physiological processes and health. This way, inulin ensures nutrition for gastrointestinal microbiota, which stimulates digestion and immune reactions (Wilson and Whelan, 2017). Inulin has antioxidant and anti-inflammatory properties (Javadi et al., 2018, Shang et al., 2018) and affects metabolism of saccharides and lipids (Rendón-Huerta et al., 2012, O'Connor et al., 2017). It stimulates laying of eggs in hens (Shang et al., 2018), therefore we cannot exclude a potential positive effect on reproductive system of humans. It mitigates symptoms of irritable bowel syndrome, Crohn's diseases (Wilson and Whelan, 2017) and lipidation of liver (Javadi et al., 2018). In patients suffering from diabetes, inulin decreased the level of insulin, cholesterol and glucose in blood, but in healthy people and patients with metabolic syndrome, these effects were not conclusively validated (Liu et al., 2017, O'Connor et al., 2017).

2.7.3. Positive Effects on Weight Reduction

Consumption of inulin creates a sensation of fullness in the gastrointestinal tract without real intake of calories by the body. Therefore, it suppresses appetite (Korczak and Slavin, 2018) and can be a calorie-free replacement for saccharides and fat in food (Majzoobi et al., 2018). Additionally, chicory (Sun et al., 2014) and inulin (Rendón-Huerta et al., 2012, Sun et al., 2014, O'Connor et al., 2017) alter gastrointestinal microbiota and stimulate the activity of bacteria in colon. These bacteria produce fatty acids, which trigger the sensation of satiety.

Feeding rats chicory extract reduced their obesity (Sun et al., 2014). Consumption of chicory inulin reduced storing of fat in quails (Lin et al., 2014). In people with obesity, inulin treatment reduced appetite and consumption (Reimer et al., 2017, Sanchez et al., 2017). In patients suffering from the early stages of diabetes, inulin reduced storing of lipids in liver and muscles and stimulated weight loss (Guess et al., 2015). In patients with liver lipidation, body weight was also reduced (Javadi et al., 2018).

Gastrointestinal microbiota was affected not just by pure inulin (see above) but also inulin in combinations with a product of its hydrolyse – oligofructose (Anastasovska et al., 2012, Sanchez et al., 2017). Determined was also inhibiting effect of pure oligofructose on appetite (Korczak and

Slavin, 2018). Oligofructosaccharides by themselves also influenced appetite also in healthy humans (Hess et al., 2011) as well as those with obesity (Sanchez et al., 2017). It is notable that the character of oligofructosaccharides' effect depends on sex: in women, it significantly suppressed appetite and food consumption, but in men this effect was small (Sanchez et al., 2017) or even converse (Hess et al., 2011). In experiments of Pol et al., (2018), consumption of oligofructosaccharides affected neither appetite nor BMI of men and women with obesity.

2.7.4. Possible Adverse Side-Effects

Claims exist that excessive chicory intake leads to the expulsion of important microelements and minerals, especially zinc, iron and calcium (https://www.nazdravie.sk/cakanka-obycajna/). Inulin can trigger flatulence, bloating, stomach and bowel noises, belching, intestinal cramping, diarrhoea, and occasionally allergic reactions (Coussement, 1999, Bacchetta et al., 2008). In the available literature, not data on adverse side-effects of fructooligosaccharides are reported.

2.7.5. General Evaluation and Recommendations

The analysis of the existing knowledge indicates applicability of chicory and its molecule inulin to suppress appetite. Aside from these effects, inulin/fructooligosaccharides can have also other positive effects on health. Adverse side-effects of inulin are not very notable and none are known for fructooligosaccharides. These data enable us to recommend inulin as a preparation intended to limit appetite and stimulate weight loss. Unlike inulin and oligofructosaccharides, sweet products of inulin's hydrolyse had in some cases no effect on appetite (Pol et al., 2018), or their effect was not significant (Sanchez et al., 2017). In another experiment, in men fructooligosaccharides did not suppress appetite, but in fact stimulated it (Hess et al., 2011) and did not facilitate weight loss (Pol et al, 2018).

Therefore, unlike inulin, we do not recommend use of oligofructosaccharides to stimulate weight loss.

2.8. FLAXSEED (*LINUM USITATISSIMUM* L.)

2.8.1. Introduction: Provenance and Properties

Flaxseed or linseed (*Linum usitatissimum L.*) is a plant from the *Linaceae* family. The earliest evidence of flaxseed products comes from approximately the 7th century BC from Iran. Cultivated flaxseed reached Europe approximately 4 thousand years later (discovery in the Switzerland). The wild predecessor of flaxseed remains unknown. Cultivated flaxseed can be divided from the economic standpoint: flax for linen, for oil, or for oil and linen.

Seed of oil flax contains 30-45% fat (drying oil whose main components are unsaturated acids – linoleic and linolenic acids), 20-30% protein, 8% water and up to 28% soluble and insoluble fibre. In seedcoat, the soluble fibre creates gel, which can swell to multiple times its size. The seed contains 1% cyanide glycosides, of which the best-known are lignans with phytoestrogenic properties as well as high content of E vitamin (Singh et al., 2011, Martinchik et al., 2012, Parikh et al., 2018, http://www.liecive. herba.sk/index.php/koncentraty/herbar/1443-lan-siaty, https://sk.wikipedia.org/wiki/Ľan_siaty).

2.8.2. Positive Effects on Human Health

Herbarium of medicinal plants (http://www.liecive.herba.sk/index.php/koncentraty/herbar/1443-lan-siaty) repots the following therapeutic effects of flaxseed:

For the valuable properties of its gel, flaxseed is used as a treatment against constipation and to stimulate bowel activity, treat stomach irritation, stomach ulcers and to prevent stomach cancer, for bronchitis and inflammations of urinal tract.

Pressing ripe flax seeds produces flax oil. It is applied internally as well as externally. The oil is used in dermatology. Isolated esters of linoleic and linolenic acids are applied in medicinal cosmetology as ingredients in regenerative preparations.

It is very well applicable in treatment of skin diseases, burns, and as regenerative cosmetic preparation for regular skin treatment.

Some authors (Bukovský, 2009, Rhee and Brunt, 2011, Singh et al., 2011, Akhtar et al., 2013, Ren et al., 2016, Parikh et al., 2018) report preventive and therapeutic effects of molecules present in flaxseed on the occurrence of the following diseases:

- Arteriosclerosis and ischemic disease of hearth (reduces overall cholesterol, LDL cholesterol and triacylglycerols, it has antioxidant and antithrombotic effects. Active molecule: Alpha-linoleic fatty acid, lignans, phenolic acids, E vitamin, folic acid)
- Tumours. Active molecule: alpha-linoleic fatty acid, lignans, gamma tocopherol (E vitamin), folic acid (B9 vitamin), magnesium, phenolic acid, flavonoids
- Hypertension. Active molecule: alpha-linoleic fatty acid
- Type II diabetes. Active molecule: alpha-linoleic acid, lignans, gamma tocopherol (E vitamin), lignans, fibre
- Immunity stimulation. Active molecule: alpha-linoleic acid, lignans, and gamma tocopherol (E vitamin)
- Treatment of autoimmune disorders (psoriasis, systemic lupus erythematosus, asthma, rheumatoid arthritis, etc.). Active molecule: alpha-linoleic fatty acid.
- Beneficial effect on metabolism of gallic acids. Active molecules: fatty acids, fibre.
- Beneficial influence on health and hygiene of colon and maintenance of gastrointestinal microbiota. Active molecule: fibre, E vitamin, lignans, vitamins and minerals.

- Improves memory. Active molecule: omega-3 fatty acids.
- It has anti-inflammatory effects. Active molecule: omega-3 fatty acids, lignans.
- It prevents chemical intoxication. Active molecules: omega-3 fatty acids, fibre, lignans.

In addition to that, lipids, B vitamins and minerals in flaxseed help maintain healthy hair and skin – reduce redness and flaking, treat acne and eczema. Flaxseed can serve as a substitute for flour containing gluten for those, who struggle with celiac disease (https://www.webnoviny.sk/7-dovodov-preco-by-sme-mali-konzumovat-lanove-semienka/).

2.8.3. Positive Effects on Weight Reduction

Fatty acids in flaxseed reduced production of obesity stimulators in hypothalamus of rats and mice (Cintra et al., 2012). Feeding rats flaxseed meal decreased the levels of fatty acids in their blood, the size of their adipose cells, but not the feed intake or body weight (Ribeiro et al., 2016). In humans, flaxseed consumption mitigated some manifestations of obesity (inflammation, insensitivity to glucose and insulin (Rhee and Brunt, 2011)) and reduced digestibility of lipids (Kristensen et al., 2008). However, that was the extent of flaxseed's promising effect on obesity. Three groups of scientists did not determine its effect on body weight and BMI of humans (Kristensen et al., 2008, Wu et al., 2010, Rhee and Brunt, 2011). Fourth team published an article on weight reduction of people linked to flaxseed consumption (Cassani et al., 2015), but they withdrew it after a year. Therefore, the collected data indicates a possible ability of flaxseed to affect lipid metabolism, but it does not reduce body weight and obesity in animals or humans.

2.8.4. Possible Adverse Side-Effects

No adverse side-effects were determined in consumption of flaxseed products at therapeutic doses. However, when large doses are ingested, we cannot exclude possible intoxication by hydrogen cyanide, which the seeds release during milling. Therefore, the maximum recommended dose for adults are 2 table spoons of crushed flaxseed a day (http://www.liecive.herba.sk/index.php/koncentraty/herbar/1443-lan-siaty). Long-term use of flaxseed at therapeutic doses is not recommended without medical supervision in these cases: intestinal blockage, acute appendicitis, pancreatitis, peritonitis, acute painful hernia. Pregnant women should opt for flaxseed oil rather than milled flaxseed – the oil does not contain lignans with phytoestrogenic effect, which could trigger complications in pregnancy. These possible dangers, however, have not been validated by experiments and flaxseed products can be considered safe. U.S. Food and Drug Administration (FDA) considers flaxseed products considers flaxseed products safe for nursing women and nutrition of children (Drugs and Lactation Database, 2006).

2.8.5. General Evaluation and Recommendations

Flaxseed products can be a functional food with added value to prevent and treat some diseases. Whole flaxseed soaked in water or sprinkled over other food, however, provides the body only with fibre. Milled seed provides all flaxseed ingredients and flax oil (cold pressed) – its fatty acids. It is necessary to remember that also milled seeds and pressed oil, even when stored in a cool and dark place, oxidise in contact with air and therefore lose their antioxidants over a few days. It is also impossible to expect that flaxseed will be efficient for weight loss.

2.9. GARCINIA CAMBOGIA

2.9.1. Introduction: Provenance and Properties

Garcinia cambogia (*Garcinia gummi-gutta*, Halabar Tamarind) is a tropical fruit native to Indonesia. Its fruit is reminiscent of pumpkins in shape, but its size is closer to that of an orange. *Garcinia* has been used for many centuries in India, Thailand and other countries of Southeast Asia as a fruit and spice as well as a medicinal plant in traditional Asian medicine. It is an ingredient in some types of Indian and Thai curry. The peel of the fruits is high (around 60%) in hydroxycitric acid (HCA), which could be responsible for the main benefits of *Garcinia* in weight loss. In addition to HCA, it contains polyphenols, luteolin, kaempferol, xanthones (carbogiol), benzophenones (garcinol) and amino acids (gamma-aminobutyric acid) (Jana et al., 2002, Yamada et al., 2007).

2.9.2. Positive Effects on Human Health

In addition to reducing the levels of body fat (see further) and glucose in blood (Shara et al., 2003, Saito et al., 2005, Fassina et al., 2015), *Garcinia* extract and HCA have anti-diabetic, anti-inflammatory, and anti-carcinogenic effects, act against parasites and protect the liver from alcohol damage (Shivashankara et al., 2012, Semwal et al., 2015).

Kaempferol and glucosides from *Garcinia* have antioxidant, anti-inflammatory, antibiotic, anti-carcinogenic, cardio- and neuroprotective effects. They can prevent oxidative stress, diabetes and osteoporosis, as well as act against pain and allergies (Calderón-Montaño et al., 2011, 2012).

2.9.3. Positive Effects on Weight Reduction

HCA can improve lipid metabolism and lower the levels of triacylglycerols and blood cholesterol (Shara et al., 2003, Saito et al., 2005, Fassina et al., 2015). There is existing knowledge about several mechanisms of this effect. It is assumed that HCA increases the levels of serotonin – neuromediator of happiness, which can suppress the centre of hunger in brain. It inhibits the enzyme ATP-citrate lyase, which participates in the synthesis of fatty acids, triacylglycerols and cholesterol, and thus suppresses lipogenesis and accumulation of fat in the body (Semwal et al., 2015). Existing knowledge supports its ability to release and burn fatty acids from fat stores in the body and reduce blood sugar levels (Shara et al., 2003, Saito et al., 2005, Fassina et al., 2015, https://garsin.sk/?gclid=EAIaIQobChMI0qSMo6nH3gIVjIKyCh00xg0fEAAYASAAEgKZ6PD_BwE).

Studies on laboratory animals and humans demonstrated the ability of HCA to reduce appetite, body weight and production of fat, as well as to affect the metabolism of lipids (Shara et al., 2003, Saito et al., 2005, Fassina et al., 2015). Some clinical tests confirmed that *Garcinia* extract or HCA can reduce body weight of people with obesity (Preuss et al., 2004, Roongpisuthipong et al., 2005, Kudiganti et al., 2015, Maia-Landim et al., 2018). However, many clinical studies also found little (Onakpoza et al., 2011) or no influence of this treatment on body weight (Heymsfield et al., 1998, Mattes and Bormann, 2000, Jana et al., 2002, Pittler and Ernst, 2004, Opala et al., 2006, Igho et al., 2008), appetite (Mattes and Bormann, 2000) and the concentration of triacylglycerols in blood (Opala et al., 2006, Hayamizu et al., 2008). Many people with obesity or overweight people in various countries use commercial products containing *Garcinia cambogia* to improve physical shape or for self-medication. However, data on the efficiently or consequences of this usage are lacking in literature.

2.9.4. Possible Adverse Side-Effects

Some clinical studies determined no statistically significant differences in the mortality and morbidity in animals and humans using *Garcinia* and HCA products (Márquez et al., 2012). Other studies showed that people consuming *Garcinia* extract suffered from digestive issues 2 times more than those who did not consume it (Onakpoza et al., 2011). Use of *Garcinia* juice can trigger acidosis (Wong and Klemmer, 2008), nausea, stomach irritation, diarrhoea, headaches, vertigo, dry mouth, manic mental states (https://www.rxlist.com/consumer_garcinia/drugs-condition.htm) and degeneration of testicles. An adverse effect of *Garcinia* products on liver has been proven. Due to this effect, medication containing these preparations has not been approved in the USA, Canada and most EU countries (Lobb, 2009, Crescioli et al., 2018, Kothadia et al., 2018). It is not recommended to consume *Garcinia* products in combination with medication against diabetes, asthma, and blood coagulation (https://en.wikipedia.org/wiki/Garcinia).

2.9.5. General Evaluation and Recommendations

Garcinia cambogia and its molecules – HCA and kaempferol – can have many physiological effects and therefore in theory, they could be applicable as medication or food supplements. Consumption of *Garcinia* at a dose 500 mg of 50% HCA (https://spalovace-tukov.heureka.sk/atp-hca-garcinia-cambogia-100-tabliet/specifikace/#section), 800 – 1000 mg of 50% HCA (https://www.rxlist.com/consumer_garcinia/drugs-condition.
htm), 2.4 g (Mattes and Bowmann, 2000), 2.8 g (Preuss et al., 2004) or 3 g of pure HCA (Hezmsfield et al., 1998, https://www.mirapa.cz/hca-pravda-o-garcinia-cambogia-kyselina-hydroxicitronova/) can be efficient against obesity and some other diseases.

However, because *Garcinia cambogia* was inefficient in half of the clinical test, is considerably toxic, which can lead to metabolic, mental, and reproductive disorders as well as disorders of the gastrointestinal tracts, it was not tested on people without obesity and because its application is not recommended by medical agencies in developed countries, its use to facilitate weight loss is not desirable.

2.10. GINGER (*ZINGIBER ZERUMBET* L.)

2.10.1. Introduction: Provenance and Properties

Ginger *(Zingiber officinale)* originally comes from Asia, where its cultivation in India and warmer regions of China has been described as early as 2000 years ago. Nowadays it is grown in Africa, Brazil and Jamaica. Ginger is used as a medicinal plant and a spice. So far, approximately 60 biologically active metabolites – primarily polyphenols and terpenoids – have been isolated and identified in ginger (Haque and Jantan, 2017). Ginger is rich in minerals, iron, potassium, calcium, magnesium, sodium and phosphor, vitamins B3 and B6, choline and inositol, hydrocarbons α-zingiberene, ar-curcumene, β-bisabolene and β-sesquiphellandrene, essential oils and capsaicin, which is present also in *Capsicum spp.* Of polyphenols, the best-known and most biologically active are beta-hydroxy ketones gingerols and shaogoals. Gingerols are present primarily in fresh roots. Shaogoals are dehydrated derivates of gingerol, which are formed in the root during drying (Sharifi-Rad et al., 2017,
https://www.sciencedirect.com/topics/medicine-and-dentistry/gingerol
https://vysetrenie.zoznam.sk/cl/1000649/1500889/Oblubeny-zazvor-nie-je-pre-vsetkych--Vyvarujte-sa-ho-skor--ako-vam-ublizi-)

2.10.2. Positive Effects on Human Health

Ginger has been used for a long time in Chinese and Ayurvede medicine and Tibb-Unami as well as in the European traditional, alternative and classic medicine. Doctors recommend application of ginger to treat arthritis and rheumatoid arthritis. It has anti-inflammatory and analgesic effects, helps to treat inflamed and dislocated joints, pain, cramping, constipation and digestive difficulties, nausea, hypertension, dementia, fever, infectious diseases and helminthiasis. It stimulates urination and prevents bloating (Chrubasik et al., 2005, Ali et al., 2008, Saldanha et al., 2016, Haque and Jantan, 2017, https://primar.sme.sk/c/6808809/zazvor-je-zdravy-viac-ako-styri-gramy-denne-vsak-neuzivajte.html#ixzz5Vcx7Bndu) Ginger has beneficial effects on digestion, nausea (for example during pregnancy or travel) and is efficient against cough and cold. It stimulates blood circulation as well as heart activity, and it even acts as an aphrodisiac (https://www.biopoint.sk/p/165/zazvorovy-prasok-500g?gclid=CjwKCA jwyOreBRAYEiwAR2mSkjNOg-MbfTFQ0zvQEJVDI3T3jJEYVH-_G359Rm4YgcajcWgDjyC-PxoCQRQQAvD_BwE). Ginger and its antioxidant components have anticancer and anti-inflammatory effects, prevents programmed cell death (apoptosis) and decreases levels of insulin and sugar in blood, which means it can be efficient in treatment of diabetes (Semwal et al., 2015, Taghizadeh et al., 2017, Zhu et al., 2018, Maharlouei et al., 2019), oxidative stress and bowel syndrome (Banji et al., 2014).

Essential oils of ginger have antimicrobial effects. One of ginger's molecules – zerumbone – has antioxidant and anti-inflammatory properties. It inhibits differentiation of cancer cells and their repletion and it decreases the vitality of tumours (Kalantari et al., 2017).

Gingerols and shaogoals are also applicable as medication to treat cancer, diabetes, heart and liver diseases (Semwal et al., 2015). Gingerol has similar chemical composition to capsaicin, which is the molecule causing the hot taste of peppers (see earlier). Gingerols and shaogoals have an effect similar to that of acetylsalicylic acid. They reduce blood coagulation, improve its circulation and therefore contribute to protection of the cardiovascular system.

2.10.3. Positive Effects on Weight Reduction

Data on the effect of ginger on levels of lipids – triglycerides – and cholesterol in blood are contradictory. Some publication reports the ability of ginger to reduce levels of cholesterol and lipids in blood (Semwal et al., 2015, Kalantari et al., 2017, Taghizadeh et al., 2017). Other experiments (Mansour et al, 2012, Pourmasoumi et al., 2018, Maharlouei et al., 2019) determined no effect of ginger consumption on most markers of lipid metabolism. In studies by Maharlouei et al. (2019), ginger even increased the levels of HDL cholesterol.

Likewise, the information on the character and mechanisms of ginger's action on body weight are contradictory. Ginger reduced body weight in animals, but the data about its effect on humans are contradictory and often negative (Ebrahimzadeh Attari et al., 2018). For example, some studies demonstrated ginger's ability to reduce weight (Mansour et al., 2012, Taghizadeh et al., 2017, Maharlouei et al., 2019). In other experiments, ginger did not facilitate weight loss (Roberts et al., 2007. Ebrahimzadeh Attari et al., 2018). Even in the experiments of Greenway et al (2006), weight loss due to ginger's influence was less notable than that in the control group. In his experiments, ginger at small doses led to an increase in body weight.

Regarding the possible mechanisms of action, it is presumed that ginger can cause weight loss by:

- increasing fat oxidation and dissipation of heat (Mansour et al.,2012, Saravanan et al., 2014),
- reducing rate of production and storing of fat (Mansour et al.,2012, Saravanan et al., 2014),
- inhibiting lipid absorption in intestines (Ebrahimzadeh Attari et al., 2018),
- suppressing appetite (Wang et al., 2017, Ebrahimzadeh Attari et al., 2018),
- delaying faecal output (Banji et al., 2014)

However, all these phenomena were validated only partially and some experiments did not validate them at all. For example, in the studies of Banji et al., (2014), ginger was activated by antioxidant enzymes and did not increase but instead decreased fat oxidation in rats. Ginger had almost no effect on healthy colon mucus membrane (Stoner, 2013). In one study on rats (Mansour et al., 2012) and one on humans (Saravanan et al., 2014), ginger enhanced the thermogenic effect of food, but other studies (Greenway et al., 2006; Gregersen et al., 2012), did not confirm this effect. When it comes to suppressing appetite, the results are similar. In the experiments of Mansoura et al. (2012) ginger suppressed it, but in other studies (Greenway et al., 2006, Roberts et al., 2007, Gregersen et al., 2012) ginger consumption had no measurable effect on appetite. In the experiments of Greenway et al., (2006) ginger at small doses in fact stimulated appetite. Therefore, the character and mechanisms of ginger's action on body weight remain unknown and further studies are required.

2.10.4. Possible Adverse Side-Effects

Clinical observations indicate some toxic side-effects of ginger (Chrubasik et al., 2005, Haque and Jantan, 2017). Ginger should be avoided by people who suffer from blood circulation disorders (particularly haemophilia), because ginger improves and stimulates blood circulation, which means it can lead to excessive bleeding in these patients. It might affect diabetic and anticoagulation treatment. It might cause nausea, vertigo, vomiting, intestinal issues, respiratory issues, pounding heart, flatulence, irritation of stomach and oral cavity (https://vysetrenie.zoznam.sk/cl/1000649/1500889/Oblubeny-zazvor-nie-je-pre-vsetkych--Vyvarujte-sa-ho-skor--ako-vam-ublizi-, https://feminity.zoznam.sk/c/894853/zazvor-a-jeho-ucinky-zazrak-v-malom-mnozstve#ixzz5VdFVo4Yk).

2.10.5. General Evaluation and Recommendations

Ginger and its molecules might have a positive effect on various physiological processes and health. The doses of ginger which had a physiological effect in previous studies were 500 mg (Greenway et al., 2006, Saldanha et al., 2016), 1000 mg (Saldanha et al., 2016), 2000 mg (Mansour et al., 2012), 2800 mg (Saldanha et al., 2016) or 1800-5000 mg Saravanan et al., 2014). Even relatively low doses (250 mg) of ginger, stimulated appetite rather than suppressed it as predicted (Greenway et al., 2006). Therefore, the dose of ginger which could lead to weight loss should be between 500-5000 mg.

Just like hot peppers, ginger at this high efficient dose could too spicy and unpalatable to consumers. Therefore, processing methods are being developed (fermentation, steaming with or without consequent dehydration, frying or "aging") to treat ginger before its use in order to mitigate its taste and aroma but not the content of the beneficial components (Choi, 2019).

Application of ginger to reduce body weight, regardless of dosage, should be considered an open question. Results of research of its effect on fat and weight loss are contradictory. Dosage is not determined. Mechanisms of its actions are not clear and the data on them are also contradictory. Therefore, its application to facilitate weight loss cannot be considered justified. In conclusion, if you enjoy ginger in food or beverages, use it. However, you cannot expect it to make you thinner.

2.11. *HOODIA GORGONII*

2.11.1. Introduction: Provenance and Properties

Hoodia (*Hoodia gordonii*) is a succulent plant similar to cactus, which grows in South African desert Kalahari. It contains steroid glycosides 3beta-[beta-D-thevetopyranosyl-(1-->4)-beta-D-cymaropyranosyl-(1-->4)-beta-D-cymaropyranosyloxy]-12beta-tigloyloxy-14beta-hydroxypregn-5-en-20-

one (1) and 3beta-[beta-D-cymaropyranosyl-(1-->4)-beta-D-6-thevetopyranosyl-(1-->4)-beta-D-cymaropyranosyl-(1-->4)-beta-D-cymaropyranosyloxy]-12beta-tigloyloxy-14beta-hydroxypregn-5-en-20-one (van Heerden et al., 2007). Commercial extract of Hoodia contains a mixture of these glycosides, fatty acids, phytosterols and alcohols (Scott et al., 2012).

2.11.2. Positive Effects on Human Health

In addition to suppressing appetite (see further), it can act on the hormones of pancreas and lower the levels of sugar in blood and internal organs. In animals, glycoside from Hoodia p57 stimulated production of glycogen in pancreas, which regulates blood sugar (Tsoukalas et al., 2016). Research of other scientists showed that the active molecule of *Hoodia gordonii* is not p57 but instead another steroid glycoside – gordonoside F – which influences insulin production and thus carbohydrate metabolism (Zhang et al., 2014).

2.11.3. Positive Effects on Weight Reduction

The scientific data on Hoodia's active molecules and mechanisms of action on body weight are contradictory. Steroid glycoside p57, isolated from *Hoodia gordonii*, when injected into the brain, was able to repress appetite in rats. This effect could have been caused by increased level of adenosine triphosphate in the hypothalamic centre responsible for appetite (MacLean and Luo, 2004). However, later studies performed on mice determined that p57 is rapidly degraded in mouth and does not reach the brain (Madgula et al., 2010). Therefore, it is unlikely to be the primary active molecule of Hoodia suppressing appetite (Smith and Krygsman, 2014b).

Research of other scientists showed that the active molecule of *Hoodia gordonii* is another steroid glycoside gordonoside F, which decreases the consumption of food in mice (Zhang et al., 2014). Other studies determined that Hoodia extract can directly reduce the number and size of fat and muscle cells and trigger degenerative chances inside them. These observations brought the authors to the conclusion that weight loss under the influence of Hoodia is caused only by an unspecific damage to cells by Hoodia toxins (Smith C, Krygsman, 2014b).

Substances in Hoodia were capable of reducing weight of animals but not of humans. Steroidal glycosides in Hoodia when fed to rats (MacLean and Luo, 2004, van Heerden et al., 2007) and rabbits (Dent et al., 2012) suppressed their appetite as well as weight. Clinical tests of Hoodia's effect on appetite and weight loss in humans, however, showed negative results. Bloom et al. (2012) found no influence of Hoodia extract on these parameters in women with obesity. Based on the fact that no information exists about the precise composition of the commercial Hoodia products (some of them contained no Hoodia molecules at all) and because there is a lack of knowledge from studies carried out on humans, in Canada (Whelan et al., 2010) and the USA (Smith and Krygsman, 2014b) it is not recommended to sell them or use them as medication or supplements. Pharmaceutic company Pfizer ceased development of weight loss products based on Hoodia p57. Food company Uniliver also stopped the development of Hoodia-based weight loss products due to the health risks and lack of efficacy (https://en.wikipedia.org/wiki/Hoodia_gordonii).

2.11.4. Possible Adverse Side-Effects

Experiments on rats showed that Hoodia extract can reduce the volume of the muscle mass (Smith C, Krygsman, 2014a). Mutagenetic actions of Hoodia on cells (Scott et al., 2012) or reproduction (Dent et al., 2012) were not determined. Clinical tests demonstrated that consumption of Hoodia products can lead to nausea, vomiting, increased skin sensitivity, hypertension, increased pulse rate, increased level of bilirubin and alkaline phosphatase in blood (Blom et al, 2012), which can be a proof of negative effect on the central nervous, cardiovascular and gastrointestinal systems.

Existing data demonstrates liver damage caused by Hoodia (https://en.wikipedia.org/wiki/Hoodia_gordonii).

2.11.5. General Evaluation and Recommendations

Previous research demonstrated the ability of *Hoodia gordonii* extract and molecules to positively influence metabolism of carbohydrates and to reduce fat and body weight of laboratory animals (mice, rats) with the help of various mechanisms of action. However, an effect of *Hoodia gordonii* extract and molecules on metabolism and weight loss in humans has not been proven. At the same time, *Hoodia gordonii* can pose a danger to health. Therefore, I do not recommend the use of Hoodia for humans.

I cannot exclude that extracts from other *Hoodia* varieties could be even more efficient than those of *Hoodia gordonii*. For example, *Hoodia parviflora* does not have the same toxic (Lynch et al., 2013) and adverse side-effects on health (Landor et al., 2015). It reduced appetite and body weight of women (Landor et al., 2015). However, the other varieties of *Hoodia* are even less explored than *Hoodia gordonii*. Therefore, I consider their application premature as well.

2.12. *IRVINGIA GABONENSIS*

2.12.1. Introduction: Provenance and Properties

Irvingia gabonensis (also known as wild mango, African mango, bush mango, dika or ogbono) grows and is cultivated in the countries of West Equatorial Africa for its fruit and seeds. Its juicy and sweet fruit contains 15.7% of carbohydrates, 0.9% protein, 0.2% fat, phosphor, calcium, iron and a large amount (70 g/kg) of C vitamin. The seeds are rather calorie dense (6 970 cal/kg). They are high in fat (67%), primarily in the form of myristic acid, lauric acid, oleic acid, palmitic acid and stearic acid. These belong to saturated fatty acids. At the same time, they contain 15% carbohydrates,

8.5% proteins, calcium and iron (Tchoundjeu Z, Atangana, 2007). Other authors (Sun and Chen, 2012) identified in the seeds of African mango high levels of ellagic acid and its glycosides – antioxidants with anti-tumour effect (Ceci et al., 2018). *Irvingia gabonensis* oil is resistant to high temperatures and oxidation, therefore it can be used as a replacement for palm oil and other oils used in the food industry (Zoué et al., 2013). *Irvingia* oil has considerable antioxidant abilities as well (Ojo et al., 2018).

2.12.2. Positive Effects on Human Health

It has antibacterial (Fadare and Ajaiyeoba, 2008) and antiparasitic (Nweze et al., 2013) effects. It can reduce pain (Okolo et al., 1995). In African medicine, *Irvingia* is used to treat neurodegenerative disorders. It is probable that its antioxidants can suppress oxidative stress, which can be a cause for these disorders (Ojo et al., 2018). *Irvingia gabonensis* can neutralize the toxic effect of cadmium on kidneys (Ojo et al., 2014) and arsenic on liver (Gbadegesin et al., 2014). *Irvingia gabonensis* extract inhibits bowel movements, which indicates it is suitable for application as a natural diarrhoea treatment (Abdulrahman et al., 2004).

Fibre form *Irvingia gabonensis* suppressed the absorption of glucose in the intestines of rats (Omoruyi and Adamson, 1993). In humans, *Irvingia gabonensis* decreased the concentration of blood sugar, therefore it was successful in treatment of diabetes (Adamson et al., 1990) and metabolic syndrome (Ngondi et al., 2005, 2009, Oben et al., 2008, Méndez-Del Villar et al., 2018).

2.12.3. Positive Effects on Weight Reduction

Irvingia gabonensis extract was able to suppress bowel movements of laboratory animals (Abdulrahman et al., 2004) and the activity of the transmitters regulating production and storing of fat in adipose tissue of rats (Oben et al., 2008). These experiments, carried out on animals, indicate that the molecules in *Irvingia gabonensis* can suppress the storing of fat in the body and thus reduce obesity by at least three pathways:

- retention of food in the intestines (Abdulrahman et al., 2004) and consequently triggering the sensation of satiety and a full stomach
- reducing rate of absorption of nutrients in the gastrointestinal tract (Omoruyi and Adamson, 1993) and
- repressing production and accumulation of fat in the body (Oben et al., 2008).

The fat contained in *Irvingia gabonensis* seeds did not influence the body weight of rats or the weight of their organs, although in males it reduced the weight of the liver (Nangue et al., 2011). Numerous studies confirm the ability of *Irvingia gabonensis* to facilitated weight reduction and treat obesity in humans (Ngondi et al., 2005, 2009, Oben et al., 2008, Egras, 2011, Ross, 2011, Onakpoya et al, 2013, Méndez-Del Villar et al., 2018). However, the shortcomings in the methodology of these tests cast doubt on the reliability of their results (Egras, 2011).

2.12.4. Possible Adverse Side-Effects

When applying *Irvingia gabonensis*, adverse side-effects such as headaches and sleep disorders were determined (Onakpoya et al, 2013). No toxic effects of *Irvingia*, even at large doses, were found (Kothari et al., 2012).

2.12.5. General Evaluation and Recommendations

The ability of extracts from *Irvingia gabonensis* seed to normalise metabolism of saccharides and lipids and to facilitate weight loss has been validated by experiments on animals and clinical studies on humans. Additionally, these molecules have also other medicinal and therapeutic effects. At the same time, no data exist about a significant adverse effect. Therefore, the use of *Irvingia gabonensis* extract is recommended to manage obesity and body weight of humans.

Data from the scientific literature indicate the applicability of *Irvingia gabonensis* seed extracts to stimulate weight loss of people, despite the high fat content. Utilization of *Irvingia* fruits also has potential, as they contain molecules similar to those found in the seeds but are less calorie-dense and have a pleasant fruity taste, therefore they could be used also to flavour and sweeten food.

2.13. KONJAC (*AMORPHOPHALLUS KONJAC* K. KOCH) AND ITS MOLECULE GLUCOMANNAN

2.13.1. Introduction: Provenance and Properties

Konjac (*Amorphophallus konjac, K. Koch*, synonyms *A. rivieri* a *A. paeoniifolius*) belongs to the *Araceacea* family. It is grown as an edible plant in South and Southeast Asia and on the islands in the Indian Ocean. It attracts attention from public because its root/bulb comprises approximately 40% glucomannan – polysaccharide soluble in water, which acts as fibre in the body. It has very low energy value. Glucomannan is characterised by excellent water-binding capacity and ability to produce gel and absorb saccharides, proteins and cholesterol. It is difficult to digest by human enzymes but processed by gastrointestinal microbiota, which makes it a prebiotic (Keithley and Swanson, 2005, Singh et al., 2018, Vollmannová et al., 2018, https://www.healthline.com/nutrition/glucomannan#weight-loss, https://www.webmd.com/vitamins/ai/ingredientmono-205/glucomannan , https://en.wikipedia.org/wiki/Konjac). Konjac has been in use for 5000 year in China, Japan and Southeast Asia as an ingredient for cooking as well as in Asian folk medicine. Thanks to its scent reminiscent of fish, it is popular in vegan cuisine as well (Chua et al., 2010, https://en.wikipedia.org/wiki/Konjac).

2.13.2. Positive Effects on Human Health

Glucomannan can play a role in reducing glucose values to treat Type II diabetes. It mitigates symptoms of the metabolic syndrome and the related cardiovascular diseases. General medical practitioners claim it relieves also hypertension, constipation and increased activity of thyroid (Keithley and Swanson, 2005, Ho et al., 2017, https://www.namaximum.sk/kategoria/zdrave-potraviny/glucomannan-konjac-glukomanan/#100-g/, https://www.webmd.com/vitamins/ai/ingredientmono-205/glucomannan, https://www.webmd.com/vitamins-supplements/ingredientreview-205-glucomannan.aspx?drugid=205&drugname=glucomannan). Traditional Chinese medicine uses glucomannan to detoxify the body, suppress growth of tumours, lower blood pressure, remove mucus, treat asthma and hernia, and counter pain, inflammation and certain types of blood and skin diseases (Chua et al., 2010). So far, scientific studies have not validated these effects.

2.13.3. Positive Effects on Weight Reduction

Glucomannan lowers levels of cholesterol and triacylglycerols in blood and lipids in the body (Keithley and Swanson, 2005, Ho et al., 2017) through several mechanisms. Glucomannan increases the volume of stomach content without an increase in calorie intake. It absorbs nutrients (saccharides, proteins and cholesterol) and therefore prevents their absorption in the gastrointestinal tract. All of that suppresses the activity of the brain centre of hunger, suppresses hunger and consequently the need to consume food and promotes weight reduction (Burton-Freeman, 2000, Keithley and Swanson, 2005). Reduced weight after intake of 2-4 g of glucomannan was determined in adult patients suffering from obesity (Keithley and Swanson 2005, Sood et al., 2008, Zalewski et al., 2015). Critical analysis of the relevant publications by other authors (Onakpoya et al., 2014), however, did not determine a definitive and statistically significant positive effect of glucomannan on body weight in adults with obesity.

Rogovik and Goldman (2009) published data on successful application of glucomannan in treatment of adolescent patients with obesity, where it enhanced the effect of orlistat, the only medication approved for treatment of adolescent obesity. The data on results of obesity treatment in children, however, are insufficient to evaluate glucomannan application in children (Zalewski et al., 2015). However, Sood et al., (2008) reported that treatment of obese child patients was less successful than that of adults.

Despite the marketing campaigns promoting glucomannan as a weight loss product for everyone, in the available literature there are no scientific data on its effect in people who are not being treated for obesity.

2.13.4. Possible Adverse Side-Effects

In case of insufficient water intake, glucomannan might not reach the stomach and due to its absorption abilities, it can then obstruct the respiratory and gastrointestinal tracts (https://www.namaximum.sk/kategoria/zdrave-potraviny/glucomannan-konjac-glukomanan/#100-g/). Some existing publications suggest glucomannan can create discomfort in the gastrointestinal tract and cause diarrhoea or constipation (Onakpoya et al., 2014). It can cause issues to people with gluten allergy (suffering from the celiac disease) (https://www.webmd.com/vitamins-supplements/ingredientreview-205-glucomannan.aspx?drugid=205&drugname=glucomannan) and people with reduced glucose metabolism (Sood et al., 2008). In combination with diabetes medication, it can reduce blood glucose to dangerously low levels. Glucomannan is not recommended to pregnant and nursing women and to children, because its effect on these categories of people was not yet explored thoroughly (Sood et al, 2008, https://www.webmd.com/vitamins/ai/ingredientmono-205/glucomannan).

2.13.5. General Evaluation and Recommendations

Glucomannan, in addition to improving metabolism and absorption of lipids, proteins and carbohydrates, and to its prebiotic effect, and reduction of appetite and body weight, can have many more positive physiological effects. Despite the inconclusive data on its efficacy, consumption of 10 g of glucomannan a day can have merit (Keithley and Swanson, 2005, Sood et al., 2008, Onakpoya et al., 2014, https://www.namaximum.sk/kategoria/zdrave-potraviny/glucomannan-konjac-glukomanan/#100-g, https://www.webmd.com/vitamins-supplements/ingredientreview-205-glucomannan.aspx?drugid=205&drugname=glucomannan). Despite that, its efficiency in weight reduction is sometimes questionable, it is possible to recommend it as an ingredient in food with added value or weight loss beverages.

Its use in weight reduction is limited by the following factors:

- Some studies highlight its applicability as a medication to treat adult obesity, but there are no scientific data on its efficiency for prevention or weight reduction in healthy people.
- Its consumption is not recommended for adolescents, children, pregnant and nursing women.
- Its adverse side-effects and contraindications have to be taken into account.

2.14. MULBERRY (*MORUS* SPP.)

2.14.1. Introduction: Provenance and Properties

There are 24 species and more than 100 varieties of mulberry, which belongs to the *Moraceae* family. The best-known are white mulberry (*Morus alba L*), black mulberry (*Morus nigra L.*) and red mulberry (*Morus rubra L.*) (Zhang et al., 2018). Black mulberry comes originally from the region spanning from Syria to Iran and Afghanistan, while white mulberry is from China. In Europe, black mulberry was valued for its fruit already in the Ancient Rome. As early as in the 1st century AC, poet Quintus Horatius Flaccus knew that "a man will pass his summers in health, who eats after breakfast mulberries picked from a tree before the sun burns." In China and later in Europe, mulberry was grown primarily as feed for silkworm. The most suitable was white mulberry with finer leaves and fewer demands for cultivation. Wood of mulberry has high energy value. Mulberry grows up to 20 meters tall. For this reason, Maria Theresa ordered its planting along the roads (https://soda.o2.sk/miesta/priroda-slovenska/zabudnute-poklady-slovenskych-zahrad-moruse/). Thanks to their high energy value, the leaves are good feed not only for the silkworm but for other livestock as well. They contain more biologically active molecules than the fruit or the root. White mulberry contains more fat (more than 1%), proteins (10 – 13%), polysaccharides, and microelements than other mulberries, black mulberry contains is the highest in the content of antioxidants, polyphenols – flavonoids, anthocyanins, benzoic acid and chlorogenic acid, alkaloids, quercetin, rutin and their analogues, which might be responsible for the medicinal properties of mulberry (Chan et al., 2016; Yuan et al., 2017; Zeni et al., 2017, He et al., 2018; Mahboubi, 2018, Zhang et al., 2018, Rodrigues et al., 2019). Chlorogenic acid, caffeine and catechins might cause physiological effects similar to coffee and tea.

2.14.2. Positive Effects on Human Health

In Asian (Japanese and Korean) traditional medicine, extracts from leaves and branches of white and black mulberry are used to treat liver diseases and diabetes, because they reduce blood sugar (Mahboubi, 2019, Rodrugues et al., 2919). Western medical research validated that the fruit and leaf extracts of *white mulberry* are efficient in preventing high blood sugar and diabetes, oxidative stress, occurrence of tumours, toxins affecting liver and kidneys, they have antibacterial and antiviral effect, stimulate immunity and blood coagulation, reduce inflammation, increase physical and brain performance, act as antidepressants, prevent cardiovascular diseases and reduce the level of lipids in blood (Chan et al., 2016, He et al., 2018, Zhang et al., 2018, Metwally et al., 2019). Molecules from the leaves and fruits of *black mulberry* stimulate the function of the intestines and act as a detoxicant, prevent oxidative stress, have antibacterial, anti-inflammatory, antitumoral, antidiabetic effects and also reduce the levels of lipids in blood and prevent liver lipidation (Lim and Choi, 2019, Rodridues et al., 2019). Extracts from *red mulberry* were able to increase the activity of antioxidation system and reduce the activity of inflammation regulators in rats (Yang et al., 2018). Juice from berries of Australian mulberry (*Morus australis Poir*) has the ability to reduce the level of cholesterol and lipids in blood and liver and influence lipid metabolism (Wu et al., 2013) (see further). It is assumed that the positive effects on health, which white mulberry (Chan et al., 2016, Mahboubi, 2019), black mulberry (Lim and Choi, 2019) and red mulberry (Yang et al., 2018) have, are due to their high content of flavonoids with antioxidation effect and therefore also protective, antiapoptotic and antimutagenic effect. Data exist that responsible for these effects might be the anthocyanins of mulberry, which affect production and effect of transcription factors regulating inflammations and metabolism (Lee et al., 2017). He et al. (2018) consider polysaccharides of white mulberry to be the key molecules preventing obesity.

2.14.3. Positive Effects on Weight Reduction

Extract from leaves and berries of *white mulberry* was able to reduce body fat and body weight of mice, hamsters (Zhang et al., 2018) and rats (Mehboubi, 2019; Metwally et al., 2019; Rodrigues et al., 2019). Similar effect on mice was found also in the fruit of Japanese mulberry (Wu et al., 2013). Sun et al., (2015) observed no impact of quercetin isolated from white mulberry's leaves on these parameters in mice. That indicates also that quercetin is not the primary active molecule of white mulberry acting on obesity.

Experiments with mulberry on humans are insufficient and their results are contradictory. In the experiments carried out by Da Villa et al., (2014), consumption of white mulberry reduced body weight and anthropocentric values of patients treated for obesity. Conversely, in the experiments of Adamska-Patruno et al., (2018), mulberry extract and a mixture of extracts from white mulberry, broad bean, and green coffee had no effect on these obesity indexes.

Extract from the fruit of *black mulberry* was able to inhibit lipase (enzymatic solvent of lipids) by pancreatic cells, but so far no studies have been published on this mulberry species to directly reduce fat stores *in vivo* (Lim and Choi, 2019).

Mulberry has the potential to reduce obesity by several pathways:

- it reduces the activity of digestive enzymes (Mahboubi, 2018),
- it inhibits differentiations of adipose cells (Mahboubi, 2018),
- it inhibits enzymes stimulating fat production (Li et al., 2919, Mahboubi, 2018),
- it stimulates conversion of white adipose cells to brown, where fat is more easily burned (Li et al., 2919),
- it regulates metabolism of stored fat (release into blood and oxidation) (Zeni et al., 2017, Mahboubi, 2018),
- it reduces absorption of saccharides (but not lipids) from blood (Zhong et al., 2006),
- it increases sensitivity to insulin, which regulates the levels of saccharides and lipids in blood (Metwally et al., 2019),
- it affects behaviour by stimulating physical activity and energy expenditure (Metwally et al., 2019).

2.14.4. Possible Adverse Side-Effects

Numerous tests of white mulberry (Mahboubi, 2018, Zhang et al., 2018) or black mulberry (Lim and Choi, 2019) products determined no negative effects on health or behaviour of animals and humans related to their consumption.

2.14.5. General Evaluation and Recommendations

Products of leaves and berries of the different mulberry species not only have high nutritional value, but they contain many molecules beneficial to health, applicable in prevention and treatment of numerous diseases, as well. At the same time, no data exists on their negative effect. The ability of the extracts of white and red mulberry to normalise production, transport and metabolism of saccharides and lipids and facilitate weight loss in laboratory animals indicates their prospective applicability in regulation of human weight. However, only two clinical studies of white mulberry extract in obesity treatment have been carried out. In one of them, mulberry was applied in a mixture with other plant products. Both studies were carried out on a small number of patients and brought contradictory results. Therefore, a broad use of mulberry in weight loss can be considered premature for now. Clinical studies on a larger scale should be carried out first.

Despite that, due to the content of beneficial biologically active molecules, their positive effect on health of animals and humans and the absence of adverse side-effects, I recommend their use as food with added value and medicinal plants. To calculate their correct dose, however, is complicated. Different species, cultivars, and plants growing under different conditions contain a very different scale of biologically active molecules at different concentrations (Chan et al., 2016, Yang et al., 2018, Lim and Choi, 2019, Mahboubi, 2019). Therefore, a dose based on the weight of the plant tissue can be only approximate. Several candidate molecules, which affect the biological effect of mulberry, does not allow to calculate a dose based only on the amount of a given substance in the preparation. Due to this, the recommended doses can differ threefold. In the experiments of Zhong et al. (2006), the metabolic effect was observed at daily consumption of tea from one gram of mulberry leaves. The company New Nordic recommends consuming 1.2 g of their preparation from white mulberry leaves (Zuccarin) a day (https://www.newnordic.ca/products/zuccarin-diet?variant=4339114934299).

In the studies of Da Villa et al., (2014), the efficient dose of white mulberry leaf extract was 2.4 g. Adamska-Patruno et al., (2018) used in their studies on humans mulberry extract at a dose 3g. Presumably based on these studies, the database WebMD (https://www.webmd.com/vitamins/ai/ingredientmono-1250/white-mulberry) recommends daily consumption of about 3g of this preparation. The database Chinese Herbs Healing (http://www.chineseherbshealing.com/mulberry-leaf/) recommends 3-9 g a day. Based on these publications, it is possible to recommend to an average consumer 1-2 g of white mulberry leaf tea a day.

2.15. OAT (*AVENA SATIVA* L.)

2.15.1. Introduction: Provenance and Properties

Common oat (*Avena sativa L.*) is a cereal from the family of *Poaceae*. The wide-spread forms of cultivated oat today *Avena sativa spp.* were cultivated from *Avena fatua*.

The region of oat's origin is West Asia and Ancient China. From there, oat spread into Central and Northern Europe. The earliest evidence of oat's occurrence comes from the Bronze Age. Oat was then a weed growing among barley. German warriors cooked it before a war campaign and the foundation of rations for Ancient Roman legionaries were oat pancakes, which would be dipped in wine. Due to its high nutritional value, oat was for many centuries a popular food not only for soldiers but for the people from lower classes and horses as well.

Its grain digests well, it has high nutritional value, balanced composition of nutrients and high content of biologically active regulatory molecules. Oat grains have the highest protein content among all cereals (11-20%). Lipids take up as much as 5-18% of the grain's volume, which is 2 to 4 times as much as in other cereals. They are of high quality – high ratio of unsaturated fatty acids. Starch content (55-60% of the grain's content) breaks down during digestion to glucose, but its digestion is slow, therefore oat products are a source of energy long and consistently released into the body and saccharides into the blood stream. Insoluble fibre (ballast materials), which is present primarily in the peels of grain (bran), represents 40% of the grain's content, which is almost as much as in rice and two thirds more than in wheat. It is not digested by the enzymes of gastrointestinal track but by the gastrointestinal microbiota. Beta-glucan is an important component of soluble nutritional fibre (2.3 – 8.5% of the grain's content).

Oats contain the most vitamins from the vitamin B group (the most B1) out of all cereals and high levels of vitamin E. The magnesium content in oat is three times higher than in other cereals, potassium twice as high than in wheat, silicon ten times as high as in wheat. It contains a lot of calcium, iron, phosphor, phytoestrogens/flavonoids and alkaloids, the content of which can represent as much as 6 % of the grain mass. Many of these molecules have antioxidant properties (Ben Halima et al., 2015, Rasane et al., 2015, Perrelli et al., 2018, http://www.krv.fapz.uniag.sk/plodiny/Ovos%20siaty.pdf, http://www.vurv.sk/fileadmin/CVRV/subory/aktivity/2013/Ovos-Noc_vyskumnika_2012.pdf).

2.15.2. Positive Effects on Human Health

Starch contained in oat is digested slowly and does not trigger rapid increase of the glycaemic index after a meal, therefore it is recommended to people suffering from diabetes. Oat is high in fat with a high ratio of unsaturated fatty acids, which have high energy value but do not trigger increase in the levels of "bad" LDL cholesterol in blood and prevent occurrence of cardiovascular diseases. It lowers blood pressure. The less digestible fibre also reduces glucose and cholesterol in blood, which treats a wide spectrum of gastrointestinal diseases and protects the mucus membrane and microbiota of the gastrointestinal tract. The soluble fibre beta-glucan is an activator of immunity, also reduces cholesterol and glucose in blood and therefore prevents manifestations of cardiovascular diseases and diabetes (Williams, 2014, Ben Halima et al., 2015, Li et al., 2016, Damsgaard et al.,

2017, Gulati et al., 2017, García-Montalvo et al., 2018, Perrelli et al., 2018, Jane, 2019, http://www.vurv.sk/fileadmin/CVRV/subory/aktivity/2013/Ovos-Noc_vyskumnika_2012.pdf).

Oat contains the same proteins as other cereals, but in comparison to them it is suitable also for people with celiac disease. Proteins that cause issues to these people, are present in oat in only small doses and do not trigger an immune response from the organism (Rasane et al., 2015, Gilissen et al., 2016).

Polyphenols and vitamins of oat have antioxidant effects, which means they bind free radicals and are good prevention against tumours. Simultaneously, they inhibit multiplication of tumour cells. They strengthen veins and reduce inflammation. Some polyphenols of oat have phytoestrogen effect and can reduce the symptoms of menopause. Calcium and vitamins help treat osteoporosis (Ben Halima et al., 2015, Perrelli et al., 2018, http://www.vurv.sk/fileadmin/CVRV/subory/aktivity/2013/Ovos-Noc_vyskumnika_2012.pdf, https://www.zdravie.sk/clanok/56489/ovos-avena-sativa-jedna-z-najzdravsich-obilnin). Consumption of oat products stimulates physical and mental performance and health. It is even linked to a decrease in general morbidity and mortality in humans (Williams, 2014). Finally, it contributes to health of teeth, hair, skin and nails (Williams, 2014, Pirrelli et al., 2018, https://www.zdravie.sk/clanok/54642/preco-vymenit-psenicu-za-ovos-a-raz). These are the best-known medical effects of the molecules contained in oat but the list is not complete.

2.15.3. Positive Effects on Weight Reduction

Feeding mice oat fibre activated molecules responsible for conversion of white adipose tissue to brown (which is easy to burn) and for fat solution (Han et al., 2017). Feeding mice starch from wholegrain oat, its beta-glucans and their mixture reduced body weight, size of adipose cells, production of molecules responsible for synthesis of lipids and conversely activated production of molecules responsible for solution of fat (Luo et al., 2018).

People who regularly consume oat products are at decreased risk of obesity (Damsgaard et al., 2017, Quatela et al., 2017). Experiments on humans demonstrated that consumption of oat products suppresses appetite (Geliebter et al., 2014), alters cholesterol content in blood and reduces body weight and waist circumference (Geliebter et al., 2014, Williams, 2014, Li et al., 2016, García-Montalvo et al., 2018, Jane, 2019). Similar effects were observed also for insoluble oat fibre (García-Montalvo et al. 2018). Consumption of another component – soluble fibre of beta-glucans – reduced waist circumference, but not body weight (Jane, 2019).

These observations indicate that oat and its component (starch and fibre) can prevent obesity by:

- slow release of energy, extending the period of satiety and suppression of appetite (Geliebter et al., 2014, Ben-Halima et al., 2015),
- stimulating conversion of white adipose tissue to brown (Han et al., 2017),
- suppressing production of molecules responsible for lipid synthesis (Luo et al., 2018),
- fibre's ability to act as a probiotic, that is stimulating the function of gastrointestinal microbiota, which regulates metabolism and obesity (Barrea et al., 2019)

2.15.4. Possible Adverse Side-Effects

In rare instances, proteins contained in oat can trigger enterocolitis (allergic inflammation of the intestine) (Nowak-Węgrzyn et al., 2017) and celiac disease when the consumption is excessive (above 20 mg/kg of body weight). Despite that, the European Commission recognised the general safety of oat and included it on the list of components permitted in food with added value (Rosane et al., 2015).

2.15.5. General Evaluation and Recommendations

Analysis of the presented scientific data proved the benefits of consumptions of oat products as food with high value as well as means of prevention and treatment of numerous diseases. The efficacy of products from oat and its components (starch and fibre) in metabolism normalisation, reduced storing of fat, stimulation of its burning, and weight and obesity reduction is validated. Positive effects manifested at daily dose of 10-100 g (in most studies 30-60g) of this cereal or 3-4.5 g beta-glucan (Williams, 2014, Jane et al., 2019). Therefore, I certainly recommend the inclusion of oat products on the menu.

2.16. PEPPERS (*CAPSICUM* SPP.)

2.16.1. Introduction: Provenance and Properties

The *Solonaceae* family comprises 20-27 *Capsicum* species, which originated in America and of which, 5 are domesticated – *C. annuum* (bell pepper), *C. baccatum* (Peruvian pepper), *C. chinense* (bonnet pepper), *C. frutescens* (tabasco pepper), *C. pubescens* ("hairy" pepper). Every species has many cultivars. The most commonly grown in our country is *Capsicum annuum*, which is divided into three categories: non-pungent sweet peppers, moderately pungent hot peppers and pungent (chilli) hot peppers. The other *Capsicum* species are represented by only pungent (chilli) hot pepper cultivars (https://en.wikipedia.org/wiki/List_of_Capsicum_cultivars). All contain carotenoids, phenols, are high in C vitamin, B6 vitamin and A vitamin, and minerals – iron, magnesium, phosphor, potassium, and calcium. One pepper can cover the daily C vitamin requirements (Baenas et al., 2019, https://en.wikipedia.org/wiki/Capsicum). The molecules contained in *Capsicum* have strong antioxidation properties (Srinivasan, 2014). Characteristic for *Capsicum* is high content of phenylamine alkaloid s – capsaicinoids and capsinoids. Those are the secondary metabolites of *Capsicum*, most likely intended to protect the plant from herbivores and fungi. Capsaicinoids stimulate nerve endings of receptors which recognize pain or irritation caused by chemicals or burns. Molecular foundation of capsaicinoids' effects lies in their molecular bonds to specific capsaicin or also vanilloid receptors, which belong to the nociceptors perceiving hot taste. Vanilloid receptors function as ion channels for the entry of calcium ions into neurones and are opened by molecules of the capsaicin type or a heat stimulus. Painful burn caused by capsaicin triggers an inflammation – redness of the tissue and localised increase of temperature similar to the reaction to a light burn. At the same time, capsaicinoids and capsinoids can affect the central and peripheral sympathetic nervous system through an action on production of neurohormones and neuromediators (serotonin and somatostatin) (Rollyson et al., 2014, Fernandes et al., 2016, Srinivasan, 2016, Varghese et al., 2017, http://chillichilli.sk/stiplavost/kapsaicin-).

2.16.2. Positive Effects on Human Health

Antioxidation properties of *Capsicum* molecules explain their ability to prevent mutations triggered by free radicals. Thanks to the antioxidation properties, they are applicable in prevention and treatment of diseases caused by oxidative stress – atherosclerosis, diabetes, cataracts and tumours (Srinivasan, 2014, Fernandes et al., 2016).

Their ability to activate vanilloid receptors means capsaicinoids are able to stimulate blood circulation, increase metabolic rate, stimulate stomach secretion and therefore also digestion. It reduces acidity and increases secretion in the gastrointestinal tract and therefore, *Capsicum* is suitable for prevention and treatment of stomach ulcers (Srinivasan, 2016). It activates intracellular insulin and glucagon, decreases levels of blood sugar (Zhang et al., 2017) and reduces the symptoms of metabolic syndrome and diabetes (Varghese et al., 2017, Sanati et al., 2018). It improves the metabolism of carbohydrates: it redirects glycogen accumulation from the liver (where it is stored) to muscles (where it is burned) (Kim et al., 2018).

Capsaicin applied in higher doses to skin before surgeries eliminates post-operation pain. It treats neuralgic pain in muscles and joints.

Capsaicinoids have antibacterial, fungicidal and anti-inflammatory effects and therefore are also conservative. They prevent storing of cholesterol on arterial walls and damage to blood cells by cholesterol, therefore protecting the cardiovascular system (Srinivasan, 2016, https://www.ncbi.nlm.nih.gov/books/NBK459168/). On the capsaicinoid base, anti-inflammation medication and analgesics are being developed (Rollyson et al, 2014, Baenas et al., 2019). These can be used to treat arthritis, neuropathic pain, dysfunctions of the digestive tract and tumours (Rollyson et al, 2014, Fernandes et al., 2016, https://www.ncbi.nlm.nih.gov/books/NBK459168/, http://www.ncbi.nlm.nih.gov/books/NBK501824/). For its ability to reduce pain, capsaicin has a soothing effect and improves sleep (Tremblaz et al., 2016).

2.16.3. Positive Effects on Weight Reduction

In mice, feed containing capsaicin decreased fat storing in liver and levels of the adipose tissue hormone leptin (Seyithanoğlu et al., 2016). *Capsicum* extract reduced their obesity and body weight (Vieira-Brock et al., 2018). In the experiments of Zhang et al. (2017), however, capsaicin did not reduce the body weight of rats.

In humans, regular or one-time consumption of *Capsicum annuum* red pepper or capsules with its extract led to reduced appetite for fat, savoury or sweet food (Ludy and Mattes, 2011, Zanzer et al., 2018). Large-scale multicentric experiments validated that consumption of capsaicinoids reduces weight, abdominal fat stores, appetite, and food consumption. Therefore, capsaicinoids and capsinoids can be an efficient ingredient in food with added value and food supplements applicable in programmes focused on weight reduction and improvement of metabolism (Kawabata et al., 2006, Reinbach et al., 2009, Whiting et al., 2012, Clegg et al., 2013, Varghese et al., 2017).

The ability of *Capsicum* molecules to reduce fat stores can be explained by multiple mechanisms of action:

- They modify the ultrastructure of cells of the gastrointestinal tract and increase of their throughput for nutrients (Srinivasan, 2016).
- They facilitate apoptosis (programmed death) of adipose cells (Lu et al., 2018)
- They reduce the size of adipocytes (Mosqueda-Solís et al., 2018)
- They suppress activity of the enzymes responsible for production of fat in adipose tissue, consequently reducing the production (Lu et al., 2018)
- They stimulate release of catecholamines (metabolism activating hormones) into blood (Gannon et al., 2016)
- They activate conversion of white adipose tissue to brown and the enzymes responsible for oxidation and burning of fat through heat dissipation instead of its sparing in adipose tissue (Ludy and Mattes, 2011, Clegg et al., 2013, Gannon et al., 2016, Tremblay et al., 2016, Varghese et al., 2017, Lu et al., 2018, Silvester et al., 2018, Vieira-Brock et al., 2018)
- They act on the sympathetic nervous system (Varghese et al., 2017) and the reduced appetite after consumption of *Capsicum* molecules (Reinbach et al., 2009, Ludy and Mattes, 2011, Whiting et al., 2014, Gannon et al., 2016, Tremblay et al., 2016, Zanzer et al., 2018) indicates that these molecules can suppress the brain centre responsible for the sensation of hunger
- Capsaicin can have an indirect effect through its ability to reduce pain, soothe, improve sleep and consequently reduce food consumption (Treamblay et al., 2016).

2.16.4. Possible Adverse Side-Effects

Regular consumption of red pepper reduced it effect due to habit-formation (Ludy et al., 2011). At the same time, *Capsicum* or capsaicinoids can sometimes cause irritation of intestines or skin. They can also increase the risk of bleeding, therefore patients who take blood-thinning medication should be very cautious. They can trigger reaction in people allergic to plants from the *Solanaceae* family or suffering from asthma (https://www.ncbi.nlm.nih.gov/books/NBK459168/, http://www.ncbi.nlm.nih.gov/books/NBK501824/). Long-term consumption of capsaicin in large (over 100 mg/kg body weight) doses can cause stomach ulcers and facilitate occurrence of prostate, duodenum and liver cancer and metastases in breast cancer (Rollyson et al., 2014). Two occurrences of heart attack have been reported in patients taking cayenne pepper pills (Sayin et al., 2012, Akçay et al., 2017), but direct causation was not proven. Regardless of these incidents, the U.S. Food and Drug Administration generally considers *Capsicum*-based food supplements and medication safe and does not require special permits for their production and application (http://www.ncbi.nlm.nih.gov/books/NBK501824/).

2.16.5. General Evaluation and Recommendations

Extracts and components of *Capsicum* can have positive effects in prevention and treatment of multiple diseases. Experiments on animals and clinical tests demonstrated the positive effects on food intake, production and storing of fat, whereby these are performed on multiple levels of regulation. Conclusively validated was the applicability of *Capsicum* extract and its components to reduce body weight in healthy people as well as people with excess weight. Despite possible health risks, *Capsicum* is considered a safe and efficient method to suppress appetite and stimulate weight loss. It can be efficient in long-term (more than 12 weeks) as well as short-term (even one-time) application. If we are asking whether to use *Capsicum* and its molecules to stimulate weight loss, the answer is clearly "yes."

The question of how to use them has a more complicated answer. Individual tolerance to capsaicinoids can be an issue. According to the results of research, daily doses of these molecules stimulating weight loss in humans were 2 mg to 10 g (in animals as much as 100 g). Capsacinoids, however, are responsible for the hot taste of *Capsicum* and act on taste receptors at extremely low doses already. Lovers of hot food will enjoy this treatment. However, for other people consumption of hot preparations at this dosage may be unbearable. For those, less hot but just as biologically efficient pills and beverages are being tested (and might be already available for purchase) (Kawabata et al., 2006, Rollyson et al., 2014, Gannon et al., 2016, Zanzer et al., 2018, Baenas et al., 2019).

2.17. PLUM (*PRUNUS DOMESTICA* L.)

2.17.1. Introduction: Provenance and Properties

European plum (*Prunus domestica* L), as well as a related species Japanese plum (*Prunus salicina Lindl.*), is a deciduous tree from the *Rosaceae* family. European plum probably evolved from the cherry plum (*Prunus cerasifera*). It was domesticated in the region of the Caspian Sea and consumed as early as in the Neolithic Era. It is the most wide-spread plum species in the world. It has many subspecies and cultivars, which differ in colour, shape, taste and yield (https://en.wikipedia.org/wiki/Plum, http://www.whfoods.com/genpage.php?tname=foodspice&dbid=35). The pulp of its fruits belongs to healthy and functional foods with unique composition (Wallace, 2017). It is low in calories, contains less than 1 % fat, approximately 11 % carbohydrates (including the difficult-to-digest sorbitol), organic acids, digestible and indigestible fibre (pectin, fructates, hemicelluloses and cellulose) and many vitamins – C, K, beta-carotene, minerals – borate, potassium, copper. Plum pit contains cyanogenic glucosides including amygdalin, which also has biological, toxic and medicinal effects (Arjmandi et al., 2017, https://en.wikipedia.org/wiki/Plum, http://www.whfoods.com/genpage.php?tname=foodspice&dbid=35). Plum fruits contain also chlorogenic acid and sorbitol, difficult to digest saccharides, which can be used as calorie-free sweetener. It contains many polyphenols (anthocyanins), which are strong antioxidants (Stacewicz-Sapuntzakis, 2013, Morabbi Najafabad and Jamei, 2014, Igwe and Charlton, 2016).

2.17.2. Positive Effects on Human Health

Thanks to its antioxidant content, plum can suppress inflammation processes (Peluso et al., 2012, Igwe and Charlton, 2016) and improve memory (Igwe and Charlton, 2016). The presence of fibre and pectin determines the ability of plums to stimulate peristalsis of the gastrointestinal tract, loosen stool and treat constipation (Howarth et al., 2010, Attaluri et al., 2011). Despite its sweet taste, the increase of blood sugar and insulin levels after plum consumption is minimal (Stacewicz-Sapuntzakis, 2013). In rats and humans, consumptions of dried plums (prunes) or plum juice mitigated symptoms of diabetes (Utsunomiya et al., 2005, Furchner-Evanson et al., 2010). Polyphenolic antioxidants of plums can prevent liver cancer (Zhou et al., 2016). Plum can activate bone production and reduce bone-thinning, osteoporosis and occurrence of fractures in advanced age (Rendina et al., 2013, Arjmandi et al., 2017, Wallace, 2017). It can improve memory and prevent allergies (Igwe and Charlton, 2016).

Based on the presence of antioxidants in plums, it is possible to presume their prospective use in prevention and treatment of diseases related to oxidative stress – asthma, measles, colon cancer, arthritis, cardiovascular diseases and diabetes. The considerable fibre content in plum suggests its benefits in prevention of high cholesterol, colon cancer, haemorrhoids and to stimulate "good" gastrointestinal microbiota (Morabbi Najafabad and Jamei, 2014, https://sk.wikipedia.org/wiki/Slivka_dom%C3%A1ca, http://www.whfoods.com/genpage.php?tname=foodspice&dbid=35, https://www.healthline.com/nutrition/benefits-of-plums-prunes#section2). Some sources claim that plum "stimulates appetite, production of digestive juices, influences performance, acts against anxiety, causes contentment, ensures firm muscles and increases immunity of the organism" (https://sk.wikipedia.org/wiki/Slivka_dom%C3%A1ca). However, these claims have not been validated by experiments on animals or humans. In traditional Iranian medicine, plum is used to treat eye diseases (Namdar et al., 2015), but this effect has also not been validated yet by clinical studies.

2.17.3. Positive Effects on Weight Reduction

The presence of chlorogenic acid (which suppresses appetite) and sorbitol (difficult-to-digest saccharide) indicates that plum can trigger the sensation of satiety and therefore reduce fat stores (Stacewicz-Sapuntzakis, 2013). This effect was confirmed in animals. Plum juice suppresses in rats fed high-fat diet symptoms of obesity such as increased levels of lipids in blood (Utsunomiya et al., 2005), increased ratio of "bad" HDL cholesterol, its accumulation in veins and increase in body weight (Noratto et al., 2014, 2015). These effects on lipid metabolism were accompanied by increased ratio of lactobacteria and bacteria *Ruminococcacea* among gastrointestinal microbiota. It also increased production of short butyric acids, which can be beneficial in obesity reduction (Noratto et al., 2014). These observations demonstrate the ability of non-saccharide components of plum (likely polyphenols, vitamins or microelements) to prevent obesity through an effect on gastrointestinal microbiota. Simultaneously, plum components can also directly influence adipose cells. *In vitro* experiments showed that extract of Japanese plum suppressed differentiation of adipose cells, lipid production in them, and activated enzymes of their burning (Choe et al., 2018). Enzyme responsible for fat solution was activated after consumption of plum juice by rats *in vivo* (Utsunomiya et al., 2005). However, the only test carried out in humans published so far did not conclusively prove an effect of consumption of prunes on food intake, levels of lipids in blood and body weight of overweight women (Howarth et al., 2010). Therefore, despite the promising effects of plums in experiments on cells and rats, positive influence of plums on weight loss in humans has not been validated as of yet.

2.17.4. Possible Adverse Side-Effects

None of the clinical tests determined any adverse side-effects of plums on human health (Wallace, 2017).

2.17.5. General Evaluation and Recommendations

Thanks to its good composition, European plum can be considered a functional food with nutritional and health benefits. It can be beneficial for prevention and maybe also treatment of multiple diseases, although its effect on health might be exaggerated by some scientific sources. It has no adverse side-effects. It can be beneficial also in prevention and treatment of metabolic disorders (for example diabetes). It has medical effects against obesity in rats, but publication of a single study carried out in patients did not validate the effect of plum on appetite, lipid metabolism and body weight in humans. Influence of plum and its components on humans requires further research.

Therefore, it is possible to recommend intense consumption of plums and plum products (not plum brandy) as delicious, healthy food, which can contribute to health and be efficient in prevention of multiple diseases. However, the effect of plum on excess weight and obesity is not validated.

2.18. STEVIA/CANDYLEAF (*STEVIA REBAUDIANA* BERTONI)

2.18.1. Introduction: Provenance and Properties

Stevia (*Stevia rebaudiana* Bertoni) is a plant from the *Asteraceae* (*Compositae*) family. It comes from Brazil and Paraguay, where Native Americans have been using it as a sweetener for centuries. Now it is cultivated in various countries for its sweet leaves. The sweet sensation is caused by Stevia glucosides (primarily steviosid, rebaudiosides A and C and steviosid metabolite isosteviol), which accumulate in leaves, flowers and roots (Carrera-Lanestosa et al., 2017). Glucosides are stable at temperatures above 200°C as well as under changing PH and they are not fermented by digestive enzymes and gastrointestinal microbiota. This means, that Stevia is non-digestible and does not contribute any calories. Glucosides are molecules, which contain glucose monomers connected to non-carbohydrate molecules – aglycones. Glucosides of Stevia activate receptors of sweetness in tongue 30-150 times (according to other data – as much as 250-300 times) as strongly as sugar (Chatsudthipong and Muanprasat, 2009, Lemus-Mondaca et al., 2012, Momtazi-Borojeni. et al., 2017, Samuel et al., 2018, https://en.wikipedia.org/wiki/Stevia). Glucosides of *Stevia rebaudiana Bertoni* have strong antioxidant effects (Carrera-Lanestosa et al., 2017) and they inhibit replication of DNA during cell multiplication (especially cancer cells) (Rojas et al., 2018). Stevia contains also inulin and oligofructosaccharides, which serve as sustenance for the gastrointestinal microbiota (Lopez et al., 2017).

2.18.2. Positive Effects on Human Health

Consumption of Stevia reduced concentrations of insulin and glucose in blood of animals (Ahmad et al., 2018) and humans and mitigated consequences of diabetes (Chatsudthipong and Muanprasat, 2009, Anton et al., 2010, Mohd-Radzman et al., 2013, Ruiz-Ruiz et al., 2017, Samuel et al., 2018). It has antioxidant, antibacterial, antifungal (Lemus-Mondaca et al., 2012, Ferrazzano et al., 2015, Carrera-Lanestosa), anti-inflammatory, diuretic and anticarcinogenic effects. It acts against diarrhoea, hypertension and stimulates immunity (Chatsudthipong and Muanprasat, 2009, Carrera-Lanestosa et al., 2017, Lohner et al., 2017, Ruiz-Ruiz et al., 2017). Therefore, besides the effects of Stevia glucosides as sweetener, it has also a therapeutic effect on treatment of cancer, diabetes, hypertension, inflammations, cystic fibrosis, and tooth decay (Momtazi-Borojeni. et al., 2017).

In the USA, Stevia has been approved as a dietetic component since 2008, in the EU since 2011 and in Japan, it has been used as a sweetener for decades (https://en.wikipedia.org/wiki/Stevia)

2.18.3. Positive Effects on Weight Reduction

Research carried out in animals and humans indicate the potential of Stevia to reduce concentration of cholesterol in blood, fat stores and body weight (Ahmad et al., 2018, https://en.wikipedia.org/wiki/Stevia). Stevia has several mechanisms for this purpose:

- Glucosides, inulin and fructooligosaccharides of Stevia can "fool" receptors of sweetness. It triggers sensation of sweetness and satiety without an actual increase of glucose in blood (Anton et al., 2010).
- Glucosides, inulin and fructooligosaccharides of Stevia can stimulate microbiota of the colon, which can have a positive effect on carbohydrate and lipid metabolism in the body, produce short-chain fatty acids and therefore reduce appetite (Lopez et al., 2017, O'Connor et al., 2017, https://en.wikipedia.org/wiki/Stevia).
- Inulin and rebaudiosid A can fill the colon and trigger the sensation of satiety without calorie intake and therefore reduce food intake (Anton et al., 2010, Ahmad et al., 2018) and can be a substitute for calorie dense sugars and fat in food (Majzoobi et al., 2018).

However, most data on weight reduction under the influence of Stevia were collected from experiments on animals. Clinical studies on humans demonstrated only weak or a very variable effect of Stevia. Half of clinical tests with Stevia intake showed suppressed and half increased appetite. Similarly, half of the experiments demonstrated body weight reduction and half no changes or even an increase in the body weight of both adults and children (Lohner et al., 2017). Often, the short-term decrease of food intake after the use of Stevia was eliminated by the consequent compensation eating. Therefore, studies carried out on humans do not enable to conclusively confirm the ability of Stevia to facilitate weight loss (Gardner, 2014, Lohner et al., 2017).

2.18.4. Possible Adverse Side-Effects

Indications exist regarding adverse side-effects of Stevia consumption by humans – headaches, depression, altered behaviour, attention deficit, premature birth and negative effects on heart and kidneys. However, the unreliability and contradictory nature of the existing information do not allow to draw definitive conclusion about the adverse side-effects of Stevia on healthy people or people with obesity or diabetes (Lohner et al., 2017).

Stevia has the potential to suppress reproductive functions. Feeding of Stevia to male rats led to their infertility (Planas and Kucacute, 1968). Feeding Stevia to obese female rats enhanced the negative impact of obesity on their fertility (Cho et al., 2018). In hamsters, Stevia did not affect reproductive processes and growth (Yodyingyuad and Bunyawong, 1991). Effect of stevia on reproductive functions of humans has not yet been examined, but the experiments on rats indicate a possible risk for male and female reproduction and fertility.

Mutagenic, teratogenic and carcinogenic effect of Stevia and rebaudiosid A was determined *in vitro*, but not in humans *in vivo* (Geuns, 2003, Momtazi-Borojeni. et al., 2017, https://en.wikipedia.org/wiki/Stevia). No negative effect of Stevia on development (Yodyingyuad and Bunyawong, 1991) or tooth decay Ferrazzano et al., 2015) and occurrence of allergies (Urban et al., 2015).

Steviol can affect transport of medication in the body, therefore we cannot exclude the possibility that it could influence effect of medicaments (Chatsudthipong and Muanprasat, 2009).

2.18.5. General Evaluation and Recommendations

At very high doses (1-300 g daily), stevia can affect carbohydrate and lipid metabolism (Yodyingyuad and Bunyawong, 1991, Lohner et al., 2017, https://en.wikipedia.org/wiki/Stevia). The results of clinical studies, however, did not conclusively confirm the ability of Stevia to reduce appetite and facilitate weight loss in humans (Gardner, 2014, Lohner et al.,

2017). There are also indications that consumption of Stevia can possibly be a risk to fertility (Planas and Kucacute, 1968, Cho et al., 2018). Therefore, low doses of Stevia (0.25 g/l of beverage or kg of food) can be used as calorie-free sweetener, but it cannot be considered a component which will reduce appetite and support weight loss.

2.19. TEA (*CAMELIA SINENSIS* L.)

2.19.1. Introduction: Provenance and Properties

Tea tree (*Camelia sinensis L.*) is a bush or a small tree from the *Theaceae* family grown in tropic and subtropical regions around the world. In Southeast Asia, the most common cultivar is *Camellia sinensis sinensis*, in India and on Ceylon - *Camellia sinensis assamica*. The individual varieties of tea differ in their appearance, size and even the chemical composition of the leaf. For production of beverages, food, and medication, young leaves are used. The 2-3 top young leaves are considered the most tender and valuable.

The final appearance, taste and biological effects of tea beverage are decided by the method of the leaf's processing. Based on the processing method (fermentation or oxidation), teas can be divided into a number of tea types (https://referaty.aktuality.sk/popis-a-pestovanie-caju/referat-16844). Fermentation affects the taste, colour, and aroma of the tea. Some people claim fermentation is an oxidation process, but this is not entirely clear. In the production of Pu-erh, oxidation is carried out first, followed by fermentation in the presence of bacteria. Essentially, tea oxidation is oxidation of its polyphenols, which leads to chemical changes in the tea leaves and causes not only darkening of the leaves but a change in chemical composition and taste as well. Fermentation is a process in which organic substances are transformed due to activity of microorganisms. These microorganisms produce enzymes beneficial to human health and create acidic environment, which protects food from rotting and contamination by toxins. Before fermentation, leaves are let to wilt and then rolled up to release cell sap. The leaves are then fermented in the presence of oxygen at temperature around 35 °C. Fermentation is finished when the desired colour and aroma have been reached (https://botanic.sk/slovnik-pojmov/fermentace, http://www.cajovnik.sk/caj-a-jeho-druhy.html).

Based on the processing method (fermentation or oxidation) and the taste, colour, aroma and biological effect of the tea, we recognize white, green, matcha, black, oolong, and Pu-erh tea (Rothenberg et al., 2018, http://www.cajovnik.sk/caj-a-jeho-druhy.html, https://en.wikipedia.org/wiki/Camellia_sinensis).

Leaves of *white* tea are harvested before they unfurl and then they are wilted. They are dried slowly in direct sunlight. They undergo no further mechanical processing and are usually not fermented at all. Due to that, the brewed tea remains light, almost colourless.

In production of *green t*ea, the harvested tea leaves are wilted. Then they are rapidly heated to destroy the enzymes which cause fermentation. The tea is then dried in sun or in an oven and sorted. Therefore, in green tea, like in white, almost no fermentation takes place.

Matcha is green tea of high quality milled into fine powder, which is used in Japanese tea ceremony.

Black tea acquires its colour through fermentation, thanks to which tea leaves turn reddish or even dark brown and the colour of the brew ranges from honey to brown. The entire process developed in the past because tea leaves travelled a long time from the East to Europe. In Asia, non-fermented tea is preferred.

*Oolong i*s somewhere between green and black tea. It is referred to also as half-fermented or blue or blue-green tea.

Pu-erh is a tea prepared from enormous green leaves, pressed and long fermented by bacteria and fungi until it acquires reddish-brown colour. This tea is very low in tannins. Its brew is dark brown with earthy or even smoky taste. It is similar to black tea. Pu-erh is suitable for long transport, during which it matures.

Despite most of Europe and the New World being accustomed to black tea, more antioxidants and tannins are present in non-oxidated and nonfermented white and green teas (http://www.cajovnik.sk/caj-a-jeho-druhy.html) and they also have a stronger benefit on health.

From standpoint of biology and medicine, the most important are tea metabolites – alkaloid theobromine, its metabolite caffeine and polyphenols (theaflavins), catechins – epigallocatechin, epicatechin and their metabolites epigallocatechin gallate and epicatechin gallate. Gallates contain biologically active ethers of gallic acid. Tea contains also smaller amounts of other biologically active polyphenols – quercetin, kaempferol and myricetin (Zang et al., 2016, Rothenberg et al., 2018). In addition to that, it contains microelements borate, cobalt, copper, iron, manganese, molybdenite and lead (Karak et al., 2017).

Tea polyphenols have antioxidant properties, which have a protective function against oxidative stress and occurrence of cancer (Yang et al., 2016, Rothenberg et al., 2018). On the other hand, epigallocatechin gallate can produce *in vitro* free radicals and consequently lower the vitality of regular as well as cancer cells (Yang et al., 2016).

2.19.2. Positive Effects on Human Health

Polyphenols of green tea are efficient against chronic inflammatory conditions of liver, gastrointestinal tract, and against neurodegenerative diseases (Oz, 2017). Anti-inflammatory effect of polyphenols can be explained by their action on gastrointestinal microbiota, which is responsible for immune responses (Yang et al., 2016).

Tea molecules at the right ratio counteract anxiety and stress (Unno et al., 2018). A link has been determined between green tea consumption and memory of older men. It is peculiar that the memory of older women was not affected (Xu et al., 2018).

Tea catechins can have an anti-tumour effect. They inhibit multiplication of cells, trigger their apoptosis (death) and autophagy and reduce vitality of cancer cells (Singh et al., 2018). They can even enhance the therapeutic effects of medicine against tumour diseases and simultaneously mitigate their adverse side-effects (Cao et al., 2016, Bedrood et al., 2018).

Most studies carried out on animals and humans report that tea (extract from tea tree leaves) reduces manifestations of metabolic syndrome, diabetes and cardiovascular diseases (including reducing the risk of heart attack) (Yang et al., 2018). Other studies demonstrated positive effect of tea on decreasing insulin in blood, but not on the concentration of glucose, triacylglycerols, fatty acids and hormones of adipose tissue (Mielgo-Ayuso et al., 2014, Li et al., 2016). Yang et al. (2016), however, report that the reduced glucose levels in blood can be caused by the action of green tea polyphenols on glucose production in liver.

2.19.3. Positive Effects on Weight Reduction

All performed studies (with the exception of Mielgo-Ayuso et al., 2014) validated the ability of tea and its components to reduce fat stores and body weight of humans (Huang et al., 2014, Janssens et al, 2016, Li et al., 2016, Pan et al., 2016, Vázquez Cisneros et al, 2017, Rothenberg et al., 2018, Yang et al., 2016, 2018).

This effect was achieved thanks to polyphenols (Pan et al., 2016, Silvester et al., 2019). According to the existing data, epigallocatechin and caffeine from tea leaves have independent mechanisms of effect but synergic effect on weight loss (Janssens et al., 2016, Türközü and Tek, 2017, Vázquez Cisneros et al, 2017).

According to some sources, black tea polyphenols are more efficient than green tea polyphenols (Pan et al., 2016), but other authors report evidence of stronger effect of green tea (Yang et al., 2016).

It is presupposed that tea molecules reduce fat stores through several pathways (Huang et al., 2014, Pan et al., 216, Yang et al., 2016, Rothenberg et al., 2018, Silvester et al., 2018, Willem et al., 2018):

- they reduce food consumption,
- they reduce emulsion and absorption of lipids and protein in gastrointestinal system and consequently reduce calorie intake,
- they act on gastrointestinal microbiota (lacto- and bifidobacteria), which are responsible for digestion. For example, they produce short fatty acids, which increase the rate of lipid metabolism,
- they reduce lipid production,
- they stimulate conversion of white adipose tissue to brown, increase its oxidation, burning and expenditure of energy through heat production,
- they influence neuroendocrinal metabolic regulators.

However, it is necessary to taken into consideration that the effect of green tea and its molecules manifests only when large doses are consumed. Vázquez Cisneros et al. (2017) recommend a daily dose of 100-460 mg of epigallocatechin gallate + 80 to 300 mg of caffeine a day over the course of 12 and more weeks. Yang et al. (2016, 2018) recommend 3-4 cups of strong tea (600-900 mg of catechins) a day for 8 weeks minimum (Yang et al., 2018).

2.19.4. Possible Adverse Side-Effects

Tea consumption at a dose of 3 cups a day (Karak et al., 2017) or epigallocatechin gallate at a dose of 300 mg a day over the course of 12 weeks (Mielgo-Ayuso et al., 2014), or 704 mg epigallocatechin gallate a day (Hu et al., 2018) has no significant adverse side-effects. No cyto- and genotoxic, mutagenic, carciogenic and embryotoxic effects of green tea were determined either (Bedrood et al., 2018).

Consumption of tea polyphenols can have a toxic effect on liver (Mazzanti et al., 2015) especially when consumed on empty stomach (Bedrood et al., 2018), or as pills rather than a beverage (Ho et al., 2018). Some studies report the ability to caffeine to negatively affect reproductive system – damage DNA and reduce sperm capacity and prolong pregnancy (Ricci et al., 2017).

2.19.5. General Evaluation and Recommendations

Tea belongs to humankind's favourite beverages. It has plentiful positive effects on health. It is applied in prevention and treatment of a number of diseases. In Japan, green tea is added to everything including desserts and ice cream. Influence of tea on body weight reduction is conclusively validated by science. Considering its effects, it is possible to recommend it as a method of weight loss stimulation or an ingredient in food with added value. All types of tea have a positive effect on health and weight reduction. In medication, tea can be substituted by its functional components – epigallocatechin gallate and caffeine mixed at a given ratio.

However, it is necessary to remember that the effects of tea will manifest only at large doses (3-4 cups of strong tea a day, which represents 1-2 g of tea containing 100-600 mg polyphenols) and long-term use. Minimum length of the treatment is 8 weeks. For pharmaceutic and food industry and to those unused to drinking large amounts of tea, I can recommend an alternative – condensed tea or its pure components. However, in that case its adverse side-effects on liver and reproductive system cannot be eliminated.

2.20. VELD GRAPE (*CISSUS QUADRANGULARIS* L.)

2.20.1. Introduction: Provenance and Properties

Cissus quadrangularis L. knowns also under the synonym *Cissus cactiformis Gilg.* or commonly as veld grape belongs to the family *Vitaceae* (grapes). It is a succulent vine native to Bangladesh, India and Shri Lanka. It grows or is cultivated also in Southeast Asia, Africa, Arabia, Brazil and the USA as a medicinal plant or a decorative potted succulent. The plant contains several biologically active molecules: steroids, phytosterols ($\Box$-

sitosterol), flavonoids, stilbenes and their derivates (quadrangularins A, B and C), iridoids, triterpenoids, derivates of gallic acid and resveratrol. The plant is rich also in C vitamin, carotene and calcium. These molecules have estrogenic and antioxidant properties (Stohs and Ray, 2013, Williamson, 2003, https://en.wikipedia.org/wiki/Cissus_quadrangularis, http://www.toxicology.cz/modules.php?name=News&file=article&sid=446), which have been validated experimentally (Malika and Shyamala, 2005, Oben et al., 2006, Aswar et al., 2010, Chidambaram and Carani Venkatraman, 2010).

2.20.2. Positive Effects on Human Health

The aboveground part of *Cissus quadraangularis* has been used since Ancient times by folk healers and in Ayurveda medicine to prevent and treat fractures, soothe pain, treat infections, haemorrhoids, menstrual difficulties, asthma and other diseases (Stochs and Ray, 2013, https://en.wikipedia.org/wiki/Cissus_quadrangularis, http://www.toxicology.cz/modules.php?name=News&file=article&sid=446). Modern scientific experiments demonstrated the efficacy of *Cissus quadraangularis* in treatment of majority of these diseases, and even further health benefits have been discovered. It has been validated that *Cissus* is able to treat bone fractures and decrease pain in bones (Sawangjit et al., 2016). Oestrogens in *Cissus* stimulated sexual activity (Aswar et al., 2010) and acted against osteoporosis in rats (Potu et al., 2009) and humans (Mishra et al., 2010). Experiments on animals determined its ability to mitigate pain, treat stomach ulcers caused by helicobacter as well as aspirin and indomethacin (Mishra et al., 2010). It reduces inflammation markers in human blood (Oben et al., 2006). The ability of *Cissus* molecules to bind free radicals (Chidambaram and Carani Venkatraman, 2010, Mallika and Shyamala, 2010) determines its protective effects against liver damage by oxidation (Chidambaram and Carani Venkatraman, 2010) and it can be efficient also against other toxic substances, radiation and cancer. It can reduce blood sugar in people suffering from overweight or obesity, which means it can mitigate the manifestations of metabolic syndrome and diabetes (Oben et al., 2006, 2008).

2.20.3. Positive Effects on Weight Reduction

Cissus quadrangularis was able to reduce lipidation of liver in rats (Chidambaram et al., 2010). Treatment of obese people and people with excess weight using preparations from *Cissus quadrangularis* by itself or in combination with *Irvingia gabonensis* (see above) led to reduced levels of lipids, total and LDL cholesterol in their blood and caused weight loss (Oben et al., 2006, 2008). Combination with *Irvingia gabonensis* acted better than *Cissus* by itself (Oben et al., 2008). These effects on obesity can be explained by the ability of *Cissus quadrangularis* molecules to stimulate burning of fat and dissipation of energy in the form of heat (Chidambaram et al., 2010, Stochs and Badmaev, 2016). However, the ability of this plant to facilitate weight loss was determined in two experiments carried out by the same group of scientists. Simultaneously, the majority of these data was gained when *Cissus* was used in combination with other plants and not as pure extract. Therefore, the ability of *Cissus quadrangularis* to reduce fat stores and stimulate weight reduction requires further validation by further independent studies (Sawangjit et al., 2017). Its wide use in weight reduction and treatment of other metabolic diseases is considered premature (https://www.verywellhealth.com/the-benefits-of-cissus-quadrangularis-88623).

2.20.4. Possible Adverse Side-Effects

Producers of food supplements containing *Cissus quadrangularis* report possible adverse side-effects in their use such as headaches, nausea, dry mouth, insomnia, extremely low levels of blood sugar, for which application of *Cissus* can be responsible (https://sk.simpleaslife.com/20118-side-effects-of-caffeine-free-hydroxycut.html, https://www.verywellhealth.com/the-benefits-of-cissus-quadrangularis-88623). However, clinical tests of *Cissus quadriangularis* have not validated significant adverse side-effects on physical and mental health of adults (Stohs and Ray, 2013, Sawangjit et al., 2016). Therefore, this plant is considered safe (Stohs and Ray, 2013). Effect of the plant on pregnant women and children has not been tested. Moreover, its interactions with medications remain unexamined (https://www.verywellhealth.com/the-benefits-of-cissus-quadrangularis-88623).

2.20.5. General Evaluation and Recommendations

Cissus quadriangularis L. is popular in traditional and Ayurveda medicine and many of its positive effects on physiological state and fitness have been validated by scientific experiments. Therefore, it has the potential to improve health, increase resistance against damaging factors, and to treat metabolic and other disorders including overweight and obesity. Adverse side-effects are negligible. First effect of treatment according to Oben et al., 2006, 2008, Sawangjit et al., 2017 can be observed in 4, maximum 10, weeks of treatment. However, so far too few information confirming the efficacy of *Cissus quadriangularis* in weight loss and treatment of other health issues. Therefore, advertisement and wide use of *Cissus quadriangularis* should be considered premature despite the broad offer of preparations with its extracts available for purchase.

2.21. YACÓN (*SMALLANTHUS SONCHIFOLIUS* POEPP.)

2.21.1. Introduction: Provenance and Properties

Yacón (*Smallanthus sonchifolius* Poepp.= *Polymnia sonchifolia* Poepp.) is a plant native to the Andes from Columbia to Argentine. Its leaves and tubers have sweet taste, because they contain inulin and the products of its hydrolysis – fructooligosaccharides. Yacón syrup contains up to 50 %

fructooligosaccharides and approximately 35 % fructose and has sweet taste reminiscent of caramelised sugar (Lachman et al., 2003, (https://en.wikipedia.org/wiki/Yac%C3%B3n). It is also rich in antioxidant (Yoshida et al., 2002).

2.21.2. Positive Effects on Human Health

It is presumed that thanks to its considerable antioxidation properties, Yacón could be applicable to neutralize polyphenolic and phenolic endocrine disruptors which contaminate the environment (Yoshida et al., 2002).

In Bolivia and Brazil, Yacón syrup is used in traditional medicine as treatment against diabetes and kidney diseases (https://en.wikipedia.org/wiki/Yac%C3%B3n). This knowledge from traditional medicine was validated also by experiments. Yacón syrup improved health, function of pancreas and carbohydrate metabolism in rats suffering from diabetes or kidney damage (Aybar et al., 2001). It did not affect blood glucose in humans (Genta et al., 2009). Likely due to its inulin content, it can improve composition of gastrointestinal microbiota and its metabolic and immune functions (Caetano et al., 2016, Cao et al., 2018).

2.21.3. Positive Effects on Weight Reduction

In Peru, Yacón syrup can be used as food that is filling despite the low-calorie content (https://en.wikipedia.org/wiki/Yac%C3%B3n). Inulin and fructooligosaccharides are really difficult to break down by enzymes of the gastrointestinal tract (Cao et al., 2018). Yacón syrup can suppress activity of intestinal pathogenic bacteria and simultaneously contribute energy to the "good" gastrointestinal microbiota, which can affect lipid and saccharide metabolism and their accumulation in the body, as well as appetite (Caetano et al., 2016, Cao et al., 2018).

In clinical tests, Yacón syrup reduced the level of LDL cholesterol (but not lipids – triglycerides) in blood, appetite and body weight of humans (Genta et al., 2009, Gomes da Silva et al., 2017). It is interesting that these changes were more notable and statistically significant only in women but not in men (Gomes da Silva et al., 2017). Existing experimental data indicates that Yacón syrup can act against obesity through:

- increasing the volume of food in intestines while calorie intake remains low,
- reducing appetite and
- an action on gastrointestinal microbiota responsible for food metabolism and other physiological processes.

2.21.4. Possible Adverse Side-Effects

In the available literature, no information could be found about adverse side-effects of Yacón syrup. However, inulin present in syrup can cause flatulence, stomach inflation, abdominal and bowel sounds, belching, intestinal cramping, diarrhoea, and occasionally allergic reactions (Coussement, 1999, Bacchetta et al., 2008).

2.21.5. General Evaluation and Recommendations

Yacón is relatively unexplored, but it has the potential to be an ingredient in functional food. Existing information indicates that Yacón syrup has multiple effects beneficial to health, for example it counters diabetes, metabolic syndrome and obesity. Therefore, its use to support weight loss can be justified.

A dose of 8-10 g a day can be enough for its physiological effect (Coussement, 1999, Bacchetta et al., 2008). Genta et al. (2007) suggest 10-20 g a day.

However, regarding its application, it needs to be taken into account that it might be efficient only in women.

2.22. YERBA MATÉ (*ILEX PARAGUARIENSIS* A.-ST.-HIL)

2.22.1. Introduction: Provenance and Properties

Yerba Maté (*Ilex paraguariensis A.-St.-Hil*), a plant from the *Aquifoliaceae* family, is wide-spread in tropical regions of South America (Southern Brazil, Northern Argentine, Paraguay and Uruguay) (Gambero and Ribeiro, 2015). It begins its development as a bush, which can grow up to 15 meters tall. From its leaves and branches, maté extract can be produced by steeping in hot or cold water. Maté consumption, as an alternative to coffee or tea, is a traditional element of social life in its native countries. Some carry containers of maté constantly and take regular sips. An average Uruguayan consumes 10 kg of Yerba Maté a year (https://en.wikipedia.org/wiki/Yerba_mate). The *Ilex* family comprises approximately 600 species. Some of them, Kudingcha (*Ilex kudingcha C.J. Tseng* and *Ilex latifolia Thunb* from China), Yaupon (*Ilex vomitoria* from the Southeast USA) and Guayusa (*Ilex guayusa Loes* from South America) can be used to produce medicinal and stimulating beverages (Gan et al., 2018). Yerba Maté, as well as its relatives, contains large amount of caffeine polyphenols, alkaloid s, tannins, and saponins (Gambero and Ribeiro, 2015, Gamboa-Gomez et al., 2015). The content of these molecules in Yerba Maté is similar to that in coffee and tea, but Yerba Maté contains more polyphenols (Gambero and Ribeiro, 2015) with stronger antioxidant capacity (de Oliveira et al., 2015, Jongberg et al., 2019) than green tea.

2.22.2. Positive Effects on Human Health

In traditional medicine, it is used as a mild stimulator of nervous system as well as a diuretic drug. Biomedicinal research validated the ability of

Yerba Maté to reduce the levels of insulin, glucose, lipids and cholesterol in blood of animals and humans (Gamboa-Gomez et al., 2015, Messina et al., 2015). Yerba Maté has antioxidant, antibacterial, anti-inflammation and antitumor properties. It prevents diseases of cardiovascular system as well as bone thinning in menopause. It improves gastrointestinal microbiota. Kudingcha, a relative of Yerba Maté, has in addition to these properties also the ability to counter diabetes and neurodegenerative diseases (Gan et al., 2018), therefore I do not exclude Yerba Maté could have this effect as well. The likely medicinal properties of Yerba Maté and its related species are explained by the presence of polyphenols and alkaloids, which have antibacterial, antioxidant, anti-inflammatory and phytoestrogenic properties (Gan et al., 2018, Balsan et al., 2019). When phenols were eliminated from the Yerba Maté extract, its ability to decrease the level of lipids in human blood was eliminated as well (Souza et al., 2017).

2.22.3. Positive Effects on Weight Reduction

Yerba Maté extract reduced obesity (accumulation of fat, levels of lipids in blood and body weight) in rats and mice (Borges et al., 2013, Gambero and Ribeiro, 2015, Gamboa-Gomez et al., 2015, Yimam et al., 2016, Gan et al., 2018).

Andersen (2001) and Fogg demonstrated reduction of body weight in patients with obesity after consuming a mixture of extracts from Yerba Maté, Guarana seeds (*Paullinia cupana*) and leaves of Damiana (*Turnera diffusa*). Other authors, however, did not report any data on changes in body weight of patients under the influence of Yerba Maté, Guarana and Damiana (Harrold et al., 2013). Kim et al. (2015) studied the effect of pure Yerba Maté extract on patients with obesity and determined reduction of fat stores, WHR and body weight. Studies by other authors did not confirm the effect of Yerba Maté consumption on body weight and other anthropometric parameters (Messina et al., 2015), levels of lipids (Souza et al., 2017) and a marker of obesity (leptin) (Balsan et al., 2019) in patients.

Action of Yerba Maté on lipid metabolism of animals and humans can be facilitated by several mechanisms. Yerba Maté is capable of:

- suppressing appetite and reducing food intake (Harrold et al., 2013, Gamboa-Gomez et al., 2015, Yimam et al., 2016). These effects are probably performed by altering the level of nonapeptide Y, which is a regulator of appetite, in brain (Gamboa-Gomez et al., 2015). Some data indicate the influence of Yerba Maté on leptin concentration in brain (Yimam et al., 2016). Other data do not validate the effect of Yerba Maté on leptin production (Gamboa-Gomez et al., 2015, Balsan et al., 2019).
- slowing the rate of food's passage through the intestines and faecal output (Andersen and Fogh, 2001).
- inhibiting the differentiation and growth of adipose cells (Gan et al., 2018).
- reducing the activity of enzymes of lipid synthesis and lipids' accumulation in adipose cells and liver (Gan et al., 2018).
- increasing burning (oxidation) of fat (Alkhatib, 2014, Alkhatib and Atcheson, 2017, Maufrais et al., 2018, Willems et al., 2018).
- increasing energy expenditure (Alkhatib, 2014, Gamboa-Gomez et al., 2015, Alkhatib and Atcheson, 2017, Gan et al., 2018, Maufrais et al., 2018).

2.22.4. Possible Adverse Side-Effects

Some performed studies determined no negative effects of Yerba Maté consumption on health of animals (de Sousa et al., 2019) and people (Andersen a Fogg, 2001, Harrold et al., 2013, Kim et al., 2015). However, known are also cases of toxic effects of consuming preparations containing Yerba Maté on humans including ischemic stroke (Lüde et al., 2016).

2.22.5. General Evaluation and Recommendations

Yerba Maté indisputably belongs into the category of efficient functional food (food with added value). It has many positive effects on health. Simultaneously, it is a promising candidate for a natural product which could be used to manage lipid metabolism and in prevention and treatment of obesity. Existing data on the effect of Yerba Maté on weight reduction are currently too few, indefinite, and contradictory. At present, the positive effect of Yerba Maté on weight loss in humans was validated only by one clinical study (Kim et al., 2016) and one successful experiment (Andersen and Fogg, 2001), in which Yerba Maté was only one component in the tested mixture. Other studies have not confirmed this effect. Therefore, clinical application of Yerba Maté on weight loss requires further validation and is premature at present.

Clinical experiments demonstrated that Yerba Maté can be efficient at a large spectrum of daily doses – 0.112 g (Harrod et al., 2013), 1 g (Alkhatib, 2014, Willems et al., 2018), 3 g (corresponding 107 mg of phenols and 84.24 mg of chlorogenic acid; Souza, 2017), 50 g or 100 g (Kim et al., 2015, Messina et al., 2015). Personally, I would recommend a daily dose of 1-2 g. Recommended is consumption of 0.5 l (Maufrais et al., 2018) to 1 l (Balsan et al., 2019) of the beverage a day. Cold Maté beverage stimulates fat oxidation and dissipation of heat more than warm (Maufrais, 2018). An extract from a fresh plant is preferable. Fermentation of the Yerba Maté plant, similarly as in black tea and oolong, leads to reduction of its antioxidation capacity (Kim and Talcott 2012).

2.23. LESS POPULAR PLANT-BASED WEIGHT LOSS SUPPLEMENTS

2.23.1. Products Not Described in the Previous Chapters

Experiments on animals and some clinical tests demonstrated that weight loss can be facilitated also by application of plant extracts and molecules which are less known and less often used by companies engaged in production and marketing of preparations intended for weight loss. Data was collected on the abilities of plants such as liquorice (*Glycyrrhiza glabra*), *Caralluma fimbriata*, bitter or Seville orange (*Citrus aurantium*) and its molecule p-synephrine, grapefruits (*Citrus paradisi*), aloe (*Aloe vera*), black elder (*Sambucus nigra*), asparagus (*Asparagus officinalis*), soy (*Glycine max*), common bean (*Phaseolus vulgaris*), *Salacia reticulata*, *Sesamum indicum*, *Lagerstroemia speciosa*, *Moringa olifera*, forskolin (an extract from *Coleous forskohlii*), ephedrine (extract from *Ephedra spp.*), Rosella – Red Sorrel (*Hibiscus sabdaroffa*), *Momordica charantia*, peony (*Penia suffruticosa*), Bofutsushosan (*Pulvis ledebouriellae compositae*), ginseng (*Panax spp.*), mormodica (*Momordica charantia*), pine extract, carotenoids, lutein and fucoxanthin, flavonoids from citruses naringin and hesperidin to suppress appetite and reduce body weight of animals and humans (Hasani-Ranjbar et al., 2009, Astell et al., 2013, Gamboa-Gómez et al., 2015, Stohs and Badmaev, 2016, Akhlaghi et al., 2017, Luís et al., 2018, Ojulari et al., 2019).

The best results of all the known plant preparations for weight loss were achieved by extracts and molecules of *Ephedra spp, Cissus quadrangularis*, ginseng, mormodica, and Bofutsushosan. Mechanisms of action of these molecules (Hasani-Ranjbar et al., 2009) are consistent with the basic mechanisms described in the Introduction and the chapter following it. It is assumed that the effect of some of these plants on appetite is due to the presence of caffeine and ephedrine, which affect the centre of satiety of the central nervous system. Ephedrine (predecessor of amphetamines) and plant preparations containing ephedrine, however, are not recommended due to their adverse psychotropic side-effects. In addition to ephedrine and caffeine, other plant molecules had not significant adverse side-effects on health (Hackman et al., 2006, Hasani-Ranjbar et al., 2009). Egras et al., (2011) describes similar abilities of chemical compounds of conjugated *linoleic acid, chitosans and pyruvates.*

For some molecules, the published data on their effects are contradictory. These contradictions can be explained by varying concentration of molecules used in the different experiments. Experiments on orange (*Citrus sinensis*) components can be used as an example. Concentrated orange juice (Vieira-Brock et al., 2018) or the polyphenol hesperidin isolated from oranges (Mosqueda-Solís et al., 2018) affected weight loss in rats positively. In studies carried out on humans, preparation from orange polyphenols reduced fat content and body weight (Dallas et al., 2008, Cases et al., 2015), but unconcentrated orange juice did not alter these parameters (Ribejro et al., 2017).

This list is incomplete. Obesity epidemic in the world leads scientists and producers to seek new plant preparations which could stop it. Therefore, the number of discovered prospective plant preparations against obesity is growing rapidly. In 2008, MUDr. P. Stanko (Stanko, 2008) reported 21 natural substances which reduce body weight. The overview by Hasani-Ranjbar et al., (2009) contains more than 70 plants tested for normalisation of lipid metabolism and obesity treatment. De Freitas and de Almeida (2017) counted 75 plant species which could have a potential for obesity treatment. Jamous et al., (2018) describe as many as 90 such candidate plants. Karri et al., (2019) increased the number of species, which could potentially be used in weight loss, up to 93. At present, it is the broadest list of plant species and substances containing molecules with the potential to affect lipid metabolism and obesity treatment. The list includes the following:

1. *Acanthopanax senticosus* (Siberian ginseng)
2. *Acanthopanax sessiliflorus*
3. *Acacia mearnsii* (Australian acacia)
4. *Actinidia arguta* (hardy kiwi)
5. *Aesculus turbinata* (Japanese horse-chestnut)
6. *Agave angustifolia (Caribbean agave)*
7. *Agave potatorum* (Butterfly agave)
8. *Alpinia officinarum* (lesser galangal)
9. *Amorphophallus konjac*
    (Amorphophallus konjac, or devil's tongue)
10. *Araucaria angustifolia* (Parana pine)
11. *Arum palaestinum* (black calla lily)
12. *Aster yomena (Kitam.)* (field aster)

13. *Benincasa hispida* (winter melon, also known as wax gourd)
14. *Betula platyphylla* (Japanese white birch or Siberian silver birch)
15. *Bos indicus* (humped cattle - zebu; the active substance is its urine)
16. *Brassica nigra* (black mustard)
17. *Calotropis procera Aiton*
18. *Camellia sinensis* (tea plant)
19. *Capsicum spp* (hot and sweet peppers)
20. *Caralluma fimbriata Wall* (cactus)
21. *Carissa carandas* (dogbane)
22. *Cassia siamea* (Senna siamea, also known as Siamese cassia)
23. *Capparis decidua* (karira)
24. *Catha edulis* (khat or qat)
25. *Celastrus regelii =Trypterigium regelii* (Regel's threewingnut)
26. *Chrysanthemum indicum* (Indian chrysanthemum)
27. *Cirsium setidens* (gondre)
28. *Citrus depressa Hayata* (shiikuwasha)
29. *Citrus unshiu* (Satsuma Mandarin)
30. *Clusia nemorosa* (Clusia)
31. *Coffea arabica* (Arabic coffee)
32. *Cosmos caudatus Kunth* (Ulam raja)
33. *Crataegus azarolus* (Mediterranean medlar or azarole)
34. *Crocus sativus* (saffron)
35. *Cudrania tricuspidata* (Mandarin melon berry)
36. *Curcuma longa* (turmeric)
37. *Dioscorea oppositifolia* (Chinese yam)
38. *Diospyros kaki* (Japanese Persimmon – kaki)
39. *Eclipta alba* (false daisy)
40. *Ecklonia cava*
41. *Eisenia bicyclis* (Arame – sea oak)
42. *Eleusine indica* (Indian goosegrass)
43. *Eugenia caryophyllus* (clove)
44. *Euphorbia supina* (Prostrate Spurge)
45. *Evodiae Fructus = E. rutaecarpa* (Evodia)
46. *Garcinia cambogia* (*Garcinia gummi-gutta*)

47. *Gardenia jasminoides* (Cape jasmine)
48. *Ginkgo biloba* (gingko - the maidenhair tree)
49. *Glycine max* , *Glycine hispida* (soybean)
50. *Glycyrrhiza uralensis* (Chinese liquorice)
51. *Griffonia simplicifolia* (*Bandeiraea simplicifolia Benth.*)
52. *Paullinia cupana* (Guarana)
53. *Gymnema sylvestre* (Gurmar)
54. *Ilex paraguariensis* (Yerba Maté)
55. *Ligularia fischeri* (gomchwi or Fischers ragwort)
56. *Limonia acidissima* (wood-apple)
57. *Lonicera caerulea* (sweetberry honeysuckle)
58. *Magnolia officinalis* (houpu magnolia or magnolia-bark)
59. *Malus hupehensis* (Tea Crabapple)
60. *Malus prunifolia* (plum-leaved apple)
61. *Malva parviflora* (Cheeseweed)
62. *Morus alba* (white mulberry)
63. *Morusaustrails poir* (mulberry)
64. *Nelumbo nucifera* Gaertn (Indian lotus)
65. *Origanum dayi* (Oregano)
66. *Oroxylum indicum* (Oroxylum – Indian trumpet flower, also known as midnight horror)
67. *Panax japonicus* (Japanese ginseng)
68. *Panax ginseng* (Asian ginseng)
69. *Panax quinquefolium* (American ginseng)
70. *Peucedanum japonicum Thunb* (coastal hog fennel)
71. *Phaseolus vulgaris* (common bean)
72. *Platycodon grandiflorum* (Chinese bellflower)
73. *Prunus salicina* (Japanese plum)
74. *Psidium guajava* (common guava)
75. *Punica granatum* (pomegranate)
76. *Radix Platycodi* (the root of Chinese bellflower)
77. *Rhizoma coptidis* (Coptidis – Huanglian)
78. *Rhus coriaria* (Sicilian sumac – tanner's sumach)
79. *Rosmarinus officinalis* (Rosemary)

80. *Salacia reticulata* (Kothala himbuktu – Salacia)
81. *Salicornia europaea* (glasswort)
82. *Salix matsudana* (Chinese willow)
83. *Salvia officinalis* (Sage)
84. *Sapindus rarak* (Sapindus – lerak or klerek)
85. *Solanum tuberosum* (potato)
86. *Swertia chirayita* (Swertia)
87. *Swietenia mahogani* (American mahogany)
88. *Tripterygium wilfordii* (thunder god vine)
89. *Vaccinium ashei* (Rabbiteye Blueberry)
90. *Vitis vinifera* (grape vine)
91. *Wasabia japonica* Matsum (Wasabi)
92. Lithospermum Erythrorhizon (purple gromwell – redroot lithospermum)
93. *Zingiber officinale* (ginger)

Some of these species are described in this monograph, other are awaiting further research. And even more plants, which could normalize lipid metabolism, are waiting to be discovered. Many of them will definitely be successfully marketed. Some of them will be also clinically tested and I hope that a portion of them will be efficient also in prevention and treatment of obesity.

Chapter 3

WHICH PLANTS ARE BEST FOR WEIGHT LOSS AND WHAT DOES IT DEPEND ON?

After reading the descriptions of all these weight loss products, a logical question can arise: All that sounds nice, but which plant is the most efficient for weight reduction?

In this case, perhaps the name of any given plant is not as important as the presence of molecules influencing weight loss. You must have noticed that various plants have a similar spectrum of molecules acting on adipose tissue. The difference lies in their amount and ratio. Concentration of the active molecules and their ratio differ not only between different plant species but also between individual plants of the same species, and even in the same plant depending on *conditions, parts of the plant and physiological state*. For example, the levels of catechins in different samples of white tea can differ 10 to 26 times. These individual differences were even larger than the differences caused by processing of the tea (difference between white and green tea) (Unachukwu et al., 2010). These differences can be caused by growing conditions, physiological state of the plant and its parts, term of harvest, etc. (Pan et al., 2018).

However, also the differences between various *plant species* can be large. In the majority of cases, Yerba Maté contains more phenols and antioxidants and has a stronger impact on the parameters of obesity and inflammation than tea (Chandra et al., 2004, de Oliveira et al., 2015, Balsan et al., 2019). Simultaneously, Yerba Maté contains 1.5 times fewer polyphenols and antioxidant effects than coffee (Baeza et al., 2018) and as much as 20 times fewer polyphenols and has a weaker effect on body fat than dark chocolate (Souza et al., 2017).

The impact of the plant fibre depends on its source, *chemical structure and physio-chemical properties*. For example, high-viscosity fibre suppresses appetite more than low-viscosity one (Wanders et al., 2011).

Also, the *method of processing* the plants influences their biochemical medicinal properties. Oxidation and fermentation reduce content of multiple biologically active molecules in tea. Therefore, white tea, green tea, matcha, black tea, oolong and Pu-erh have different contents of phenols and different antioxidant activity (Unachukwu et al., 2010, de Oliveira et al., 2015, Malongane et al., 2017). For example, the catechin content in green matcha tea is 3 to 137 times higher than that in regular green tea (Weiss and Anderton, 2003).

Conditions of extraction of the biologically active molecules from the plant are also important. Biological effect of the same plant depends also on the temperature of water used to prepare the beverage. Green tea is most efficient when brewed in 100 °C water (Pan et al., 2018) and maté when cold water is used (Maufrais et al., 2018).

Even more important can be the *type of liquid used for extraction*. The majority of plants are consumed in form of herbal tea. Water, however, is not the best extractor for all substances and polyphenols solved in water degrade relatively fast and are more difficult to absorb than the ones solved in milk. Milk protects polyphenols and their antioxidant activity better than water. Contrary to the recommendations of various websites, some scientific studies recommend to prepare tea, coffee and cocoa with milk or with addition of milk (Bhagat et al., 2019). Herbal teas prepared in water also lose their biological activity at a relatively rapid rate; therefore, they should be consumed fresh. Biological activity is retained by the tea even when used in baked goods and cakes (Unno et al., 2019). Water is not ideal as a solvent for food either. The gastrointestinal tract of humans is best suited for consumption of solid food. Food in form of liquid solutions has entered the diet of adults only recently. Therefore, saccharides solved in water are less acceptable to the body and the sensation of satiety is lesser than when saccharides from solid food are consumed (Wolf et al., 2008). This serves as another argument against the consumption of sweet sodas and fruit juices at the expense of fresh fruit.

Finally, the impact of plants and their active molecules depends also on *the condition of the organism* receiving them – the adipose tissue and regulators and the ability to react to calorie intake and plant molecules from the mechanisms of direct pathways and feedback. That was described in the beginning of this monograph.

The number of difficult to control factors which affect the success of phytotherapy means its results are hard to predict. That leads to the amount of contradictory data published in scientific literature regarding the effect of the same plant. Therefore, every treatment is something of a lottery and no one can guarantee a victory with a single ticket (in this case, a plant). We can, however, increase our chances for victory by purchasing multiple tickets – applying several plants at once. Therefore, I will dedicate the following chapters to knowledge on the relationships between various plant preparations and their combinations, which have been tested on patients with obesity.

Chapter 4

COMBINATIONS OF INDIVIDUAL PLANT MOLECULES

4.1. SIMILAR EFFECTS OF INDIVIDUAL PLANT MOLECULES

As stated in the introduction, plants and plant molecules described in this book can be divided according to the different character of their effect on body weight:

- plants, which contain few easily digestible components (monosaccharides) and a lot of the ones difficult to digest (polysaccharides, fibre), which trigger the feeling of fullness – *Chia, Garcinia cambogia, glucomannan, apple cider vinegar, inulin, Stevia, Yacon syrup*
- plant molecules which repress production, proliferation and differentiation of adipose cells or stimulate conversion of white adipose tissue into brown – *Hoodia, coffee, mulberry, sweet and hot peppers, cinnamon, plum, Yerba Maté,*
- plant components which decrease the activity of enzymes responsible for production of lipids and high levels of triacylglycerols in blood – *tea, chia, Garcinia, Irvingia, apple cider*

vinegar, coffee, mulberry, sweet and hot peppers, cinnamon, Yerba Maté and ginger,
- plant components which activate enzymes responsible for burning fat, oxidation of lipids, and production of heat from fat stores – *tea, chia, Cissus, Garcinia, apple cider vinegar, mulberry, sweet and hot peppers, cinnamon, plum, Yerba Maté, ginger*
- plant components which suppress absorption of lipids – *tea, glucomannan, Irvingia, sweet and hot peppers, ginger,*
- plant components which repress the activity of the hunger centres of brain – *tea, glucomannan, Garcinia, apple cider vinegar, sweet and hot peppers, cinnamon, Stevia, Yacón syrup, Yerba Maté, ginger,*
- plant molecules which activate sweetness receptors on tongue and thus repress the feeling of hunger without noticeable calorie intake – *inulin, Stevia, Yacón syrup,*
- plant molecules which slow down discharge from the bowels and create a sensation of satiety – *Irvingia, apple cider vinegar, Yerba Maté, ginger,*
- plant substances (saccharides, fibre) – prebiotics which support the gastrointestinal microbiota, which produce short-chain fatty acids and trigger the feeling of full stomach – *tea, inulin, coffee, plum, Stevia, Yacón syrup.*

From this list it is clear that fat stores are regulated by a number of mechanisms. At the same time, each regulator can be influenced by multiple plant preparations. Similar effects of some plants can be explained also by the similarity in the biologically active molecules they contain. For example, both *Capsicum* spp. and ginger contain the biologically active molecule capsaicin. Inulin and fructooligosaccharides are present in Yacón, Stevia and many other plants. Chlorogenic acid is present in coffee and plum and Yerba Maté, and caffeine – in coffee and tea and Yerba Maté. Most of the described plants have antioxidant characteristics and therefore they can be beneficial not only in treatment of obesity but tumours and diabetes as well (though it remains unclear how these plants – antioxidants can at the same time stimulate oxidation of lipids). Therefore, there is a large "overlap" in the molecules, actions and mechanisms of the effect various plants have on fat stores. Therefore, a use of a large amount of exotic and expensive preparations with the same effect is questionable. Information summarised in this book can help the reader select plant molecules for weight loss while avoiding an overlap in their compositions and mechanisms of their actions.

4.2. POSSIBLE INTERACTIONS OF THE INDIVIDUAL PLANT MOLECULES

Science literature contains very little data about positive or negative mutual interactions of plant molecules used to promote weight loss. However, the few existing experiments prove that individual plant molecules can stimulate (synergies) but also inhibit one another (antagonists). For example, *Irvingia gabonensis* is able to enhance the effect of *Cissus quadrangularis* on weight loss in humans (Oben et al., 2008). Conversely, capsaicin from peppers and hesperidin from citrus fruit applied individually were efficient in repressing adipocytes in rats, but their combination was inefficient (Mosqueda-Solís et al., 2018). From this it is apparent that a mutual neutralization could be possible also in other plant molecules. It is impossible to exclude that inulin, glucomannan and fibre could absorb the biologically active molecules of other plants and thus inhibit their effect.

4.3. POSSIBLE COMBINATIONS OF PLANT MOLECULES

Various combinations of plant extracts and their components were tested for application in treatment of obesity. Most of these formulations contained also the molecules described previously.

The following combinations led to reduced fat stores and body weight in overweight patients:

- combination of *rhubarb, ginger, astragalus, red sage, curcuma and gallic acid* (Greenway et al., 2006, Roberts et al., 2007),
- combination of *alkaloids of ephedra, caffeine, vitamins and omega-3 fatty acids* (Hackman et al, 2006)
- combination of *asparagus, green and black tea, guarana, mate tea and common bean* (Opala et al., 2006),
- combination of *common bean, Garccinia cambogia and yeast* (Opala et al., 2006),
- combination of *Irvingia gabonensis* and *Cissus quadrangularis* (Oben et al., 2008),
- combination of *Hordeum vulgare, Polygonatum multiforum, Dimocarpus longan, Ligusticum sinense, Lilium brownii and ginger* (preparation Slimax) (Hasani-Ranjbar et al., 2009),
- combination of *Garcinia cambogia and gurmar (Gymnema sylvestre)* (Astell et al., 2013)
- combination of *green tea, capsaicin and ginger* (Taghizadeh et sal., 2017),

The following formulations were tested on people with obesity and they affected some physiological parameters, but the publications did not contain data on positive impact of these substances on fat and body weight, or scientific literature does not exist at all:

- combination of *black, green and mulberry* tea (Zhong et al., 2006),
- combination of *capsaicin and green tea* (Reinbach et al., 2009)
- combination of *pineapple, black mulberry and plum* (Peluso et al., 2012, Miglio et al., 2014)
- combination of juices from *apple, grapes, blueberries, pomegranate, grape seeds and green tea* (Miglio et al., 2014)
- combination of *white mulberry, beans and green coffee* (Adamska-Patruno et al., 2018)
- combination of *ginger, saffron and barbary fig* (preparation Bioxyn, https://www.recenzie-plus.sk/bioxyn/)

In rats, a tested combination of *capsaicin and hesperidin* (molecules from citrus fruit) did not affect obesity and body weight despite the efficiency of the substances applied individually (Mosqueda-Solís et al., 2018) (see above). All studies, with the exception of the last one, compared a combination of mixtures to a control group; therefore, their results did not enable to identify the role, efficiency and mutual relationships of the individual ingredients of the formulations. The effect of some ingredients (pineapple, apple, grapes) on weight loss in humans has not been clinically validated (see further), but the results of these experiments allow to identify the molecules and combinations which can be applicable for prevention and treatment of obesity in humans, for development of functional food and beverages and new medical procedures.

Chapter 5

SOME MYTHS ABOUT THE EFFECT OF PLANT MOLECULES INFLUENCING BODY WEIGHT

5.1. EXAMPLES OF PLANT MOLECULES UNDESERVEDLY BELIEVED TO FACILITATE OBESITY

Media targeted coconut oil with heaps of criticism due to containing lauric acid, which behaves in the body like "bad" animal saturated fat. Such articles online were published under titles such as "Don't eat coconut oil! You can damage your own health!" (http://www.tvnoviny.sk/myzeny/1833478_zdravy-ako-bukovsky-kokosovy-olej-vseliek-alebo-lacny-klam) or "Coconut oil is a concentrate of fatty acids bad for our health" (https://fitastyl.sk/clanky/vyziva/pravda-o-kokosovom-oleji-alebo-tuku-akchcete) and "Coconut oil is simply a poison, warns a doctor. It causes serious diseases" (http://tn.nova.cz/clanek/pozor-na-kokosovy-olej-zpusobuje-nemoci-srdce-a-cev.html). Coconut oil can truly mildly increase the levels of cholesterol in blood. However, it only increases the "good" (HDL) cholesterol and not the "bad" (LDL) cholesterol and it improves their ratio in blood (Assunção et al., 2009, Cardoso et al., 2015, Eyres et al., 2016). Aside from that, lauric acid from coconut oil oxidises well, causes dissipation of energy in the form of heat, and is not accumulated in fat stores

(DiNicolantonio and O'Keefe, 2017). Clinical experiments found no adverse health effects of coconut oil. In fact, its effect on weight loss was stronger than that of its competition – sunflower and soy oil and chia seed oil (Assunção et al., 2009, Cardoso et al., 2015, Oliveira-de-Lira et al., 2018). This proves that not everything containing fat (coconut oil, chia seeds and oil) facilitates obesity. These substances can in fact support weight loss in humans by so far unknown mechanisms.

Even more often, myths and diets based on them form in relation to plants thought to aid in weight loss.

5.2. Examples of Plant Molecules Mistakenly Assumed to Help In Weight Loss

The efforts to reduce weight create pressure to produce many widely-promoted diets and foodstuffs. Their effects on health and lipid metabolism are not always validated. For example, in Europe and USA wide-spread myths exist about the weight reduction abilities of St John's-wort (*Hypericum perforatum*), dandelion (*Taraxacum officinale*), rosemary (*Rosmarinus officinalis*), Roselle (*Hibiscus sabdaroffa*), avocado, lemon, pomelo, tangerine, pomegranate, pineapple, apple, wholegrain bread, peanuts and grapes. Drinking large amounts of waters is also rumored to have similar effects (https://abc-dieta.sk/chudnutie-s-hroznom.html, www.liecive.herba.sk/index.php/rok-2011/383-4-2011/1108-rakytnik-v-receptoch-ruskej-ludovej-mediciny-2.html, https://schudnutie.peknetelo.eu/citron-pomelo-grep-mandarinka-pomaranc-chudnutie.html, https://schudnut-ako.webnode.sk/news/ako-schudnut-ovocie-vhodne-a-nevhodne-na-chudnutie-/, https://wanda.pluska.sk/chudnutie-s-ananasom-zarucene/wellness-a-fit/chudnutie/539561.html). Some websites promise "Simple miracle: Drink water with lemon for 4 days and you'll get rid of as much as 2 kilograms" (https://www.pluska.sk/zena/chudnutie/dieta-tento-tyzden/jednoduchy-zazrak-pite-vodu-citronom-4-dni-zbavite-az-2-kilogramov.html).

This information is not supported by any scientific studies carried out in humans. Some of these plant-based substances affected the metabolism of fat in laboratory animals, but clinical tests found no ability of St. John's wort, dandelion, rosemary, Roselle, flax, avocado, lemon, pomegranate or peanuts to reduce obesity and weight (Gamboa-Gómez et al., 2015, Ojulari et al., 2019).

As an example, we can look at the molecules found in seeds and peels of grapes. Some experiments on rodents demonstrated the ability of these molecules to decrease fat stores, levels of cholesterol in blood, and weight (Badavi et al., 2013, Kim et al., 2015, Mahmoudi et al., 2018), but other studies did not (Ansar et al., 2017). Extracts from grape peels and seeds were tested as a component of a mixture of plant-based substances for weight reduction in humans, but their influence on fat metabolism and reduction of weight was not proven (Irandoost et al., 2013, Miglio et al., 2014).

Flaxseed can also be used as an example. Some websites not only chose titles like "Flaxseed – help in height loss" (https://vyzivovy-poradca.sk/lanove-semienka-chudnutie/), but they provide detailed recipes for brewing it as well and they recommend drinking 4 to 5 cups of such brew a day (https://poradymosk.netlify.com/krsa-a-zdravie5/pouitie-anovhose3298). Flaxseed was included even on a medical list of substances aiding in weight loss (Stanko, 2008). However, no experiment proves its effect on weight and obesity in animals or humans (see chapter "Flaxseed").

Some plants and plant molecules (ephedrine+caffeine, *Hibiscus sabdaroffa*, *Momordica charantia*, peony *Penia suffruticosa*, Bofutsushosan *Pulvis ledebouriellae compositae*) may have reduced body weight, but had no influence on the composition and metabolism of fat in the organism (Hasani-Ranjbar et al., 2009). This fact suggests these plants have no real effect on fat stores. In some cases, the effect of these plants on weight reduction was explained by dehydration and decreased muscle volume rather than the reduction of fat stores (Zamora Navarro and Pérez-Llamas, 2013). Decreased calorie intake by reduction diets had a considerably more significant impact. For example, simply skipping breakfast stimulated weight loss much more significantly than oatmeal breakfast (Geliebter et al., 2014). Food components and special diets were often unable to sufficiently increase the effect of reduced food intake (Zamora Navarro and Pérez-Llamas, 2013). After all, even the reduction diets themselves have in most cases only temporary effects, followed by the well-known "yoyo effect." Better results in reduction of fat stores and body weight were achieved by diets in combination with increased physical activity and mental programming for a lasting lifestyle change (Robertson et al., 2014). These data suggest that a consumer should not expect miracles from beverages and food containing plant molecules that promote weight loss. These components can be useful only in combination with lower calorie intake, increased burning of calories through physical activity, and psychological motivation for such change.

Chapter 6

Conclusion: What We Learned

History of plant preparations' use in prevention of metabolic disorders is as long as that of humankind. Throughout history, people around the globe collected a lot of information and experience in regards to the utilization of local flora. Knowledge on numerous plants and their combinations that prevent accumulation of fat in the body was gathered. This knowledge is implemented in medicine world-wide: Western, Asian, Latin-American, African. Detailed description of this knowledge is beyond the capacity of one book. Meanwhile, its importance is always growing, because obesity and metabolic disorders are an increasingly large threat to health, quality of life, and longevity of people. This threat incites public interest in this topic. During the times of food shortage in the past, we developed natural self-preservation instincts. These instincts tell us: "Eat as many delicious high-calorie foods as possible and store the energy you get from them." Under the contemporary conditions of abundance and unlimited availability of food, this becomes a threat for a considerable portion of the population. Common sense tells us the exact opposite: "Limit your calorie intake and exercise to burn the excess." However, nature is often not in favour of our efforts. Many objective factors exist which regulate the mechanism of fat. The perfect equilibrium between these mechanisms ensuring metabolic stability is (for better or worse) really difficult to disrupt. This means that our efforts to limit food and exercise fail to bring the expected results. The most pleasant compromise between the instincts and common sense is to introduce into our diets foods which can improve metabolism without causing internal discomfort to their consumers.

Currently, the market offers a wide variety of diets, food supplements, detoxification procedures, and weight loss medication. The advertising hype is forced on us from every direction, promising miraculous weight loss without any effort. Fortunately for the marketers (and unfortunately for the consumers), food supplements are not strictly regulated with the goal to validate their efficiency. Many of these products have never been scientifically examined and therefore we have no idea whether they are efficient at all. Many, when tested, showed to have no effect at all, to be only partially efficient, or it would be necessary to consume exuberant amounts of them to achieve results. Some would need chemical treatment. Some are efficient only in women but not in men or children. We know almost nothing about their combinations. Therefore, do not trust advertising, especially if quick results with no effort are promised. Many substances advertised by the weight loss industry have no such effects in reality.

How many and which of them are actually useful? This monograph offers a critical analysis of the most popular plants and their components used in weight loss. Based on this detailed analysis, only 9 (43%) (tea, chicory/inulin, apple cider vinegar, coffee, konjac, oat, hot and sweet peppers, cinnamon, and Yacon) were more or less scientifically proven to have these effects. These plants and their components can be recommended for reduction of weight and fat stores. Other 57% (*Garcinia cambogia, Hoodia gordinii*, chia, *Irvingia gabonensis,* flaxseed, mulberry, carob, plum, veld grape, Stevia, Yerba Maté and ginger) show insufficient or contradictory results and need to be further clinically tested.

Out of the other 39 candidate plants and their components described in detail, for 13 (33%) no scientific proof exists about their effect on metabolism of fat and weight loss (St. John's wort, dandelion, rosemary, Roselle, avocado, lemon, pomelo, tangerine, pomegranate, pineapple, apple, wholegrain bread, peanuts, grape) or they reduced weight without any impact on the fat stores (bofutsushosan *Pulvis ledebouriellae compositae, ephedrine, Hibiscus sabdaroffa*).

I do not consider my evaluation of the natural preparations' effect on weight loss to be overly critical. Other experts, Ríos-Hoyo and Gutiérrez-Salmeán (2016), examined in detail the clinical tests of 10 recently discovered plants, which are actively advertised by marketers – beans, *Garcinia cambogia*, bitter orange (*Citrus aurantum*), *Hoodia gordonii*, forskolin, green coffee, glucomannan, beta-glucan, chitosan, Guar gum (polysaccharide from guar beans, *Cyamopsis tetragonoloba), and raspberry ketones* (*Rubus idaeus*). They came to the conclusions that none of these preparations can be conclusively considered efficient in the treatments of obesity in humans. According to the authors, the clinical tests of these preparations were either not carried out yet or they were carried out on an insufficient number of patients. Or the results were either insufficient or contradictory.

This fact may be disappointing to you, but it comes as no surprise. It is a logical outcome of the current imperfect legislative. Legally, weight loss products are not considered medication, but food. Therefore, marketers only need to label the product a "food supplement" and they do not need to guarantee its effect, perform clinical and toxicological test or apply for permits with medical regulatory bodies (Egras et al., 2011).

Based on the knowledge we collected and presented in this book, plants and their molecules can be divided into three groups:

1. Those with a conclusively proven effect on weight reduction. These are not many: tea, glucomannan, inulin, apple cider vinegar, coffee, oat, sweet and hot peppers, cinnamon, and Yacon.
   From the plants described in less detail, weight reduction ability is more or less reliably proven in coconut oil, liquorice *(Glycyrrhiza glabra L.),* bitter or Seville orange (*Citrus aurantium*), aloe (*Aloe vera*), soy (*Glycine max*) and the common bean (*Phaseolus vulgaris*).
2. Plants on which little information is known, or the information is contradictory, and plants with considerable adverse side-effects.

Therefore, currently I would not recommend their broad use in weight reduction. These are *Garcinia cambogia*, *Hoodia gordinii*, chia, *Irvingia gabonensis*, mulberry, plum, veld grape, Stevia, Yerba Maté, and ginger.

To this group belong also plants not analysed in detail in this book, for example grapefruit (*Citrus paradisi*), orange (*Citrus sinensis*), *Caralluma fimbriata*, elder (*Sambucus nigra*), asparagus (*Asparagus officinalis*), *Salacia reticulata, Sesamum indicum, Lagerstroemia speciosa, Moringa olifera, Coleous forskohlii* and its molecule forskolin, *Momordica charantia*, peony *Penia suffruticosa*, ginseng (*Panax spp.*), Momordica (*Momordica charantia*), broccoli extract, carotenoids lutein and fucoxanthin, citrus flavonoids naringin and hesperidin, linolenic acid, chitosans and pyruvates.

3. Plants known to be inefficient, whose effects likely belong into the "myth" category. These are St. John's wort, dandelion, rosemary, flaxseed, carob, avocado, lemon, pomelo, tangerine, pomegranate, apple, pineapple, wholegrain bread, peanuts, parts of grapes, or preparations which reduced weight without affecting the fat stores (bofutsushosan, ephedrine, *Hibiscus sabdaroffa*).

State of metabolism and development of metabolic disorders depends on calorie intake from food, their expenditure, and what happens to them (are they stored, burned, removed in the form of heat or excrements?). All these processes can be influenced by food with added value, containing certain plant molecules. These molecules affect accumulation of fat on three levels of regulation – (1) action on the centre of hunger in CNS, (2) action on adipocytes and (3) action on the cells and bacteria in the gut. One needs to be aware that no "miraculous" plant or diet, or food supplement, will work without some effort put in. Plants with added value, however, can help considerably in our struggle. Additionally, all the aforementioned plants – whether they aid in weight loss or not – have many other health benefits. You only need to choose well.

I assume that after reading this book, the reader will have a clearer idea about how body regulates intake and expenditure of energy, what it depends on, and how it is possible to influence your weight, shape and health, as well as which activities are an unnecessary waste of time and money. I hope that it will guide consumers in their selection of weight reduction preparations and will be helpful also to researchers, doctors, producers and marketers.

SUMMARY

This book represents a critical review of the available knowledge concerning manifestations, mechanisms, consequences and prevention of dysfunctions of metabolism of fat, as well as plant preparations which can be useful for improvement of health, and for prevention and treatment of obesity. Furthermore, we tried to provide the reader with some advice and tips to combat obesity with healthy lifestyle and selected plants. The book contains a review of recent (issued after year 2000) publications concerning plant preparations for prevention and treatment of obesity, whose efficiency was validated or not validated by scientific studies. The provenance, biologically active molecules, positive and adverse side-effects on health, influence on obesity and potential applicability of tea, chicory, *Garcinia cambogia*, *Hoodia gordonii*, chia, *Irvingia gabonensis*, apple cider vinegar, coffee, konjac/glucomannan, flaxseed, mulberry, oat, sweet and hot peppers, carob, cinnamon, plum, *Cissus quadrangularis*, *Stevia rebaudiana*, Yacon and ginger are described. In addition, less-known plants and plant molecules, as well as their combinations considered applicable for obesity treatments, are listed. The book presents also a critical review of factors, especially plants and plant molecules, affecting obesity, and it presents the most popular myths concerning their influence. It is demonstrated that more than half of the plant-based anti-obesity products available on the market are not properly clinically tested, or such tests, when performed, provided negative results. Each piece of information is supported by reference to the corresponding publication, which enables its verification.

BIBLIOGRAPHY

REFERENCES

Abdulrahman F, Inyang IS, Abbah J, Binda L, Amos S, Gamaniel K. Effect of aqueous leaf extract of Irvingia gabonensis on gastrointestinal tract in rodents. *Indian J Exp Biol*. 2004;42(8):787-91.

Abeysekera WPKM, Arachchige SPG, Ratnasooriya WD. Bark Extracts of Ceylon Cinnamon Possess Antilipidemic Activities and Bind Bile Acids *In Vitro*. *Evid Based Complement Alternat Med.* 2017:7347219.

Adamska-Patruno E, Billing-Marczak K, Orlowski M, Gorska M, Krotkiewski M, Kretowski A. A Synergistic Formulation of Plant Extracts Decreases Postprandial Glucose and Insulin Peaks: Results from Two Randomized, Controlled, Cross-Over Studies Using Real-World Meals. *Nutrients*. 2018;10(8). pii: E956.

Adamson I, Okafor C, Abu-Bakare A. A supplement of Dikanut (*Irvingia gabonesis*) improves treatment of type II diabetics. *West Afr J Med.* 1990;9(2):108-15.

Ahadi Z, Qorbani M, Kelishadi R, Ardalan G, Motlagh ME, Asayesh H, Zeynali M, Chinian M, Larijani B, Shafiee G, Heshmat R. Association between breakfast intake with anthropometric measurements, blood pressure and food consumption behaviors among Iranian children and adolescents: the CASPIAN-IV study. *Public Health.* 2015;129(6):740-7.

Ahmad U, Ahmad RS, Arshad MS, Mushtaq Z, Hussain SM, Hameed A. Antihyperlipidemic efficacy of aqueous extract of *Stevia rebaudiana* Bertoni in albino rats. *Lipids Health Dis.* 2018;17(1):175.

Akçay M, Gedikli Ö, Yüksel S. An unusual side effect of weight loss pills in a young man; acute myocardial infarction due to cayenne pepper pills. *Anatol J Cardiol.* 2017;18(4):310-1.

Akhlaghi M, Zare M, Nouripour F. Effect of Soy and Soy Isoflavones on Obesity-Related Anthropometric Measures: A Systematic Review and Meta-analysis of Randomized Controlled Clinical Trials. *Adv Nutr.* 2017;8(5):705-17.

Akhtar S, Ismail T, Riaz M. Flaxseed - a miraculous defense against some critical maladies. *Pak J Pharm Sci.* 2013;26(1):199-208.

Ali BH, Blunden G, Tanira MO, Nemmar A. Some phytochemical, pharmacological and toxicological properties of ginger (Zingiber officinale Roscoe): a review of recent research. *Food Chem Toxicol.* 2008;46(2):409-20.

Alkhatib A, Atcheson R. Yerba Maté (*Ilex paraguariensis*) Metabolic, Satiety, and Mood State Effects at Rest and during Prolonged Exercise. *Nutrients.* 2017;9(8). pii: E882.

Alkhatib A. Yerba Maté (*Illex Paraguariensis*) ingestion augments fat oxidation and energy expenditure during exercise at various submaximal intensities. *Nutr Metab* (Lond). 2014;11:42.

Amiot MJ, Riva C, Vinet A. Effects of dietary polyphenols on metabolic syndrome features in humans: a systematic review. *Obes Rev.* 2016l;17(7):573-86.

Anastasovska J, Arora T, Sanchez Canon GJ, Parkinson JR, Touhy K, Gibson GR, Nadkarni NA, So PW, Goldstone AP, Thomas EL, Hankir MK, Van Loo J, Modi N, Bell JD, Frost G. Fermentable carbohydrate alters hypothalamic neuronal activity and protects against the obesogenic environment. *Obesity* (Silver Spring). 2012;20(5):1016-23.

Andersen T, Fogh J. Weight loss and delayed gastric emptying following a South American herbal preparation in overweight patients. *J Hum Nutr Diet.* 2001;14(3):243-50.

Ansar H, Zamaninour N, Djazayery A, Pishva H, Vafa M, Mazaheri Nezhad Fard R, Dilmaghanian A, Mirzaei K, Shidfar F. Weight Changes and Metabolic Outcomes in Calorie-Restricted Obese Mice Fed High-Fat Diets Containing Corn or Flaxseed Oil: Physiological Role of Sugar Replacement with Polyphenol-Rich Grape. *J Am Coll Nutr.* 2017;36(6):422-33.

Arjmandi BH, Johnson SA, Pourafshar S, Navaei N, George KS, Hooshmand S, Chai SC, Akhavan NS. Bone-Protective Effects of Dried Plum in Postmenopausal Women: Efficacy and Possible Mechanisms. *Nutrients.* 2017;9(5). pii: E496.

Assunção ML, Ferreira HS, dos Santos AF, Cabral CR Jr, Florêncio TM. Effects of dietary coconut oil on the biochemical and anthropometric profiles of women presenting abdominal obesity. *Lipids.* 2009;44(7):593-601.

Astell KJ, Mathai ML, Su XQ. A review on botanical species and chemical compounds with appetite suppressing properties for body weight control. *Plant Foods Hum Nutr.* 2013;68(3):213-21.

Astell KJ, Mathai ML, Su XQ. Plant extracts with appetite suppressing properties for body weight control: a systematic review of double blind randomized controlled clinical trials. *Complement Ther Med.* 2013;21(4):407-16.

Aswar UM, Bhaskaran S, Mohan V, Bodhankar SL. Estrogenic activity of friedelin rich fraction (IND-HE) separated from *Cissus quadrangularis* and its effect on female sexual function. *Pharmacognosy Res.* 2010;2(3):138-45.

Atawia RT, Bunch KL, Toque HA, Caldwell RB, Caldwell RW. Mechanisms of obesity-induced metabolic and vascular dysfunctions. *Front Biosci* (Landmark Ed). 2019;24:890-934.

Attaluri A, Donahoe R, Valestin J, Brown K, Rao SS. Randomised clinical trial: dried plums (prunes) vs. psyllium for constipation. *Aliment Pharmacol Ther.* 2011;33(7):822-8.

Aybar MJ, Sánchez Riera AN, Grau A, Sánchez SS. Hypoglycemic effect of the water extract of *Smallantus sonchifolius* (Yacón) leaves in normal and diabetic rats. *J Ethnopharmacol.* 2001;74(2):125-32.

Bacchetta J, Villard F, Vial T, Dubourg L, Bouvier R, Kassaï B, Cochat P. 'Renal hypersensitivity' to inulin and IgA nephropathy. *Pediatr Nephrol.* 2008;23(10):1883-5.

Badavi M, Abedi HA, Dianat M, Sarkaki AR. Exercise Training and Grape Seed Extract Co-Administration Improves Lipid Profile, Weight Loss, Bradycardia, and Hypotension of STZ-Induced Diabetic Rats. *Int Cardiovasc Res J.* 2013;7(4):111-7.

Baenas N, Belović M, Ilic N, Moreno DA, García-Viguera C. Industrial use of pepper (*Capsicum annum* L.) derived products: Technological benefits and biological advantages. *Food Chem.* 2019;274:872-85.

Baer DJ, Rumpler WV, Miles CW, Fahey GC Jr. Dietary fiber decreases the metabolizable energy content and nutrient digestibility of mixed diets fed to humans. *J Nutr.* 1997;127(4):579-86.

Baeza G, Sarriá B, Bravo L, Mateos R. Polyphenol content, in vitro bioaccessibility and antioxidant capacity of widely consumed beverages. *J Sci Food Agric.* 2018;98(4):1397-406.

Balliett M, Burke JR. Changes in anthropometric measurements, body composition, blood pressure, lipid profile, and testosterone in patients participating in a low-energy dietary intervention. *J Chiropr Med.* 2013;12(1):3-14.

Balsan G, Pellanda LC, Sausen G, Galarraga T, Zaffari D, Pontin B, Portal VL. Effect of yerba mate and green tea on paraoxonase and leptin levels in patients affected by overweight or obesity and dyslipidemia: a randomized clinical trial. *Nutr J.* 2019;18(1):5.

Banji D, Banji OJ, Pavani B, Kranthi Kumar Ch, Annamalai AR. Zingerone regulates intestinal transit, attenuates behavioral and oxidative perturbations in irritable bowel disorder in rats. *Phytomedicine.* 2014;21(4):423-9.

Bano F, Ikram H, Akhtar N. Neurochemical and behavioral effects of *Cinnamomi cassiae* (Lauraceae) bark aqueous extract in obese rats. *Pak J Pharm Sci.* 2014;27(3):559-63.

Barrea L, Muscogiuri G, Annunziata G, Laudisio D, Pugliese G, Salzano C, Colao A, Savastano S. From gut microbiota dysfunction to obesity: could short-chain fatty acids stop this dangerous course? *Hormones* (Athens). 2019; 18(3):245-50.

Bedrood Z, Rameshrad M, Hosseinzadeh H. Toxicological effects of *Camellia sinensis* (green tea): A review. *Phytother Res.* 2018;32(7):1163-80.

Ben Halima N, Ben Saad R, Khemakhem B, Fendri I, Abdelkafi S. Oat (*Avena sativa* L.): Oil and Nutriment Compounds Valorization for Potential Use in Industrial Applications. *J Oleo Sci.* 2015;64(9):915-32.

Bhagat AR, Delgado AM, Issaoui M, Chammem N, Fiorino M, Pellerito A, Natalello S. Review of the Role of Fluid Dairy in Delivery of Polyphenolic Compounds in the Diet: Chocolate Milk, Coffee Beverages, Matcha Green Tea, and Beyond. *J AOAC Int.* 2019;102(5):1365-72.

Bhatti SK, O'Keefe JH, Lavie CJ. Coffee and tea: perks for health and longevity? *Curr Opin Clin Nutr Metab Care.* 2013;16(6):688-97.

Björck I, Elmståhl HL. The glycaemic index: importance of dietary fibre and other food properties. *Proc Nutr Soc.* 2003;62(1):201-6.

Blom WA, Abrahamse SL, Bradford R, Duchateau GS, Theis W, Orsi A, Ward CL, Mela DJ. Effects of 15-d repeated consumption of Hoodia gordonii purified extract on safety, ad libitum energy intake, and body weight in healthy, overweight women: a randomized controlled trial. *Am J Clin Nutr.* 2011;94(5):1171-81.

Blüher M. Obesity: global epidemiology and pathogenesis. *Nat Rev Endocrinol.* 2019; 15(5):288-98.

Bray GA, Smith SR, de Jonge L, Xie H, Rood J, Martin CK, Most M, Brock C, Mancuso S, Redman LM. Effect of dietary protein content on weight gain, energy expenditure, and body composition during overeating: a randomized controlled trial. *JAMA.* 2012;307(1):47-55.

Bray GA. Energy and fructose from beverages sweetened with sugar or high-fructose corn syrup pose a health risk for some people. *Adv Nutr.* 2013;4(2):220-5.

Budak NH, Aykin E, Seydim AC, Greene AK, Guzel-Seydim ZB. Functional properties of vinegar. *J Food Sci.* 2014;79(5):R757-64.

Bukovský I. *Nová miniencyklopédia prírodnej liečby* [*The new encyclopedy of natural nutrition*] AKV-Ambulancia klinickej výživy, 222 s., 2009. ISBN 9788097023003.

Burton-Freeman B. Dietary fiber and energy regulation. *J Nutr.* 2000;130(2S Suppl):272S-275S.

Caetano BF, de Moura NA, Almeida AP, Dias MC, Sivieri K, Barbisan LF. Yacon (*Smallanthus sonchifolius*) as a Food Supplement: Health-Promoting Benefits of Fructooligo saccharides. *Nutrients.* 2016;8(7). pii: E436.

Calderón-Montaño JM, Burgos-Morón E, Pérez-Guerrero C, López-Lázaro M. "A review on the dietary flavonoid kaempferol." *Mini Reviews in Medicinal Chemistry.* 2011, 11 (4): 298–344.

Camacho S, Michlig S, de Senarclens-Bezençon C, Meylan J, Meystre J, Pezzoli M, Markram H, le Coutre J. Anti-obesity and anti-hyperglycemic effects of cinnamaldehyde via altered ghrelin secretion and functional impact on food intake and gastric emptying. *Sci Rep.* 2015;5:7919.

Cao J, Han J, Xiao H, Qiao J, Han M. Effect of Tea Polyphenol compounds on anticancer drugs in terms of anti-tumor activity, toxicology, and pharmacokinetics. *Nutrients.* 2016;8(12). pii: E762.

Cao Y, Ma ZF, Zhang H, Jin Y, Zhang Y, Hayford F. Phytochemical Properties and Nutrigenomic Implications of Yacón as a Potential Source of Prebiotic: Current Evidence and Future Directions. *Foods.* 2018;7(4). pii: E59.

Cardoso DA, Moreira AS, de Oliveira GM, Raggio Luiz R, Rosa G. A cconut extra virgin oil-rich diet increases HDL cholesterol and decreases waist circumference and body mass in coronary artery disease patients. *Nutr Hosp.* 2015;32(5):2144-52.

Carlström M, Larsson SC. Coffee consumption and reduced risk of developing type 2 diabetes: a systematic review with meta-analysis. *Nutr Rev.* 2018;76(6):395-417.

Carrera-Lanestosa A, Moguel-Ordóñez Y, Segura-Campos M. *Stevia rebaudiana* Bertoni: A Natural Alternative for Treating Diseases Associated with Metabolic Syndrome. *J Med Food.* 2017;20(10):933-43.

Cases J, Romain C, Dallas C, Gerbi A, Rouanet JM. A 12-week randomized double-blind parallel pilot trial of Sinetrol XPur on body weight, abdominal fat, waist circumference, and muscle metabolism in overweight men. *Int J Food Sci Nutr.* 2015;66(4):471-7.

Cassani RS, Fassini PG, Silvah JH, Lima CM, Marchini JS. Impact of weight loss diet associated with flaxseed on inflammatory markers in men with cardiovascular risk factors: a clinical study. *Nutr J.* 2015;14:5.

Ceci C, Lacal PM, Tentori L, De Martino MG, Miano R, Graziani G. Experimental Evidence of the Antitumor, Antimetastatic and Antiangiogenic Activity of Ellagic Acid. *Nutrients.* 2018;10(11). pii: E1756.

Chan EW, Lye PY, Wong SK. Phytochemistry, pharmacology, and clinical tri als ofMorus alba. *Chin J Nat Med.* 2016;14(1):17-30.

Chandra S, De Mejia Gonzalez E. Polyphenolic compounds, antioxidant capacity, and quinone reductase activity of an aqueous extract of *Ardisia compressa* in comparison to mate (*Ilex paraguariensis*) and green (*Camellia sinensis*) teas. *J Agric Food Chem.* 2004;52(11):3583-9.

Chatsudthipong V, Muanprasat C. Stevioside and related compounds: therapeutic benefits beyond sweetness. *Pharmacol Ther.* 2009;121(1):41-54.

Chen IJ, Liu CY, Chiu JP, Hsu CH. Therapeutic effect of high-dose green tea extract on weight reduction: A randomized, double-blind, placebo-controlled clinical trial. *Clin Nutr.* 2016;35(3):592-9.

Cherniack EP. Potential applications for alternative medicine to treat obesity in an aging population. *Altern Med Rev.* 2008;13(1):34-42.

Chidambaram J, Carani Venkatraman A. *Cissus quadrangularis* stem alleviates insulin resistance, oxidative injury and fatty liver disease in rats fed high fat plus fructose diet. *Food Chem Toxicol.* 2010;48(8-9):2021-9.

Cho NA, Klancic T, Nettleton JE, Paul HA, Reimer RA. Impact of Food Ingredients (Aspartame, Stevia, Prebiotic Oligofructose) on Fertility and Reproductive Outcomes in Obese Rats. *Obesity* (Silver Spring). 2018;26(11):1692-5.

Choe WK, Kang BT, Kim SO. Water-extracted plum (*Prunus salicina* L. cv. Soldam) attenuates adipogenesis in murine 3T3-L1 adipocyte cells through the PI3K/Akt signaling pathway. *Exp Ther Med.* 2018;15(2):1608-1615.

Choi JS. Processed gingers: Current and prospective use in food, cosmetic, and pharmaceutical industry. *Recent Pat Food Nutr Agric.* 2019;10(1):20-6.

Chrubasik S, Pittler MH, Roufogalis BD. Zingiberis rhizoma: a comprehensive review on the ginger effect and efficacy profiles. *Phytomedicine.* 2005;12(9):684-701.

Chua M, Baldwin TC, Hocking TJ, Chan K. Traditional uses and potential health benefits of *Amorphophallus konjac* K. Koch ex N.E.Br. *J Ethnopharmacol.* 2010;128(2):268-78.

Cintra DE, Ropelle ER, Moraes JC, Pauli JR, Morari J, Souza CT, Grimaldi R, Stahl M, Carvalheira JB, Saad MJ, Velloso LA. Unsaturated fatty acids revert diet-induced hypothalamic inflammation in obesity. *PLoS One.* 2012;7(1):e30571.

Clegg ME, Golsorkhi M, Henry CJ. Combined medium-chain triglyceride and chilli feeding increases diet-induced thermogenesis in normal-weight humans. *Eur J Nutr.* 2013;52(6):1579-85.

Coussement PA. Inulin and oligofructose: safe intakes and legal status. *J Nutr.* 1999;129(7 Suppl):1412S-7S.

Crescioli G, Lombardi N, Bettiol A, Marconi E, Risaliti F, Bertoni M, Menniti Ippolito F, Maggini V, Gallo E, Firenzuoli F, Vannacci A. Acute liver injury following Garcinia cambogia weight-loss supplementation: case series and literature review. *Intern Emerg Med.* 2018;13(6):857-872.

Da Villa G, Ianiro G, Mangiola F, Del Toma E, Vitale A, Gasbarrini A, Gasbarrini G. White mulberry supplementation as adjuvant treatment of obesity. *J Biol Regul Homeost Agents.* 2014;28(1):141-5.

Dallas C, Gerbi A, Tenca G, Juchaux F, Bernard FX. Lipolytic effect of a polyphenolic citrus dry extract of red orange, grapefruit, orange (SINETROL) in human body fat adipocytes. Mechanism of action by inhibition of cAMP-phosphodiesterase (PDE). *Phytomedicine.* 2008;15(10):783-92.

Damsgaard CT, Biltoft-Jensen A, Tetens I, Michaelsen KF, Lind MV, Astrup A, Landberg R. Whole-Grain Intake, Reflected by Dietary Records and Biomarkers, Is Inversely Associated with Circulating Insulin and Other Cardiometabolic Markers in 8- to 11-Year-Old Children. *J Nutr.* 2017;147(5):816-24.

Darzi J, Frost GS, Montaser R, Yap J, Robertson MD. Influence of the tolerability of vinegar as an oral source of short-chain fatty acids on appetite control and food intake. *Int J Obes* (Lond). 2014;38(5):675-81.

de Almeida Paula HA, Abranches MV, de Luces Fortes Ferreira CL. Yacon (*Smallanthus sonchifolius*): a food with multiple functions. *Crit Rev Food Sci Nutr.* 2015;55(1):32-40.

de Freitas Junior LM, de Almeida EB Jr. Medicinal plants for the treatment of obesity: ethnopharmacological approach and chemical and biological studies. *Am J Transl Res.* 2017;9(5):2050-64.

de Oliveira CC, Calado VM, Ares G, Granato D. Statistical Approaches to Assess the Association between Phenolic Compounds and the in vitro Antioxidant Activity of *Camellia sinensis* and *Ilex paraguariensis* Teas. *Crit Rev Food Sci Nutr.* 2015;55(10):1456-73.

de Roos B, Sawyer JK, Katan MB, Rudel LL. Validity of animal models for the cholesterol-raising effects of coffee diterpenes in human subjects. *Proc Nutr Soc.* 1999;58(3):551-7.

de Sousa WR, Lourenço BHLB, Reis MP, Donadel G, Marques MAA, Cardozo Junior EL, Jacomassi E, Belettini ST, Lívero FADR, Gasparotto Junior A, Lourenço ELB. Evaluation of reproductive toxicology of aqueous extract of Yerba Mate (*Ilex paraguariensis* A. St.-Hil.), a traditional South American beverage. *J Med Food.* 2019;22(1):97-101.

de Souza Ferreira C, dd Sousa Fomes Lde F, da Silva GE, Rosa G. Effect of chia seed (*Salvia hispanica* L.) consumption on cardiovascular risk factors in humans: a systematic review. *Nutr Hosp.* 2015;32(5):1909-18.

Dempersmier J, Sambeat A, Gulyaeva O, Paul SM, Hudak CS, Raposo HF, Kwan HY, Kang C, Wong RH, Sul HS. Cold-inducible Zfp516 activates UCP1 transcription to promote browning of white fat and development of brown fat. *Mol Cell.* 2015;57(2):235-46.

DiNicolantonio JJ, O'Keefe JH. Good Fats versus Bad Fats: A Comparison of fatty acids in the promotion of insulin resistance, inflammation, and obesity. *Mo Med.* 2017;114(4):303-7.

Dionísio M, Grenha A. Locust bean gum: Exploring its potential for biopharmaceutical applications. *J Pharm Bioallied Sci.* 2012;4(3):175-85. doi:10.4103/0975-7406.99013.

Doepker C, Franke K, Myers E, Goldberger JJ, Lieberman HR, O'Brien C, Peck J, Tenenbein M, Weaver C, Wikoff D. Key Findings and implications of a recent systematic review of the potential adverse effects of caffeine consumption in healthy adults, pregnant women, adolescents, and children. *Nutrients.* 2018;10(10). pii: E1536.

Dorri M, Hashemitabar S, Hosseinzadeh H. Cinnamon (*Cinnamomum zeylanicum*) as an antidote or a protective agent against natural or chemical toxicities: a review. *Drug Chem Toxicol.* 2018;41(3):338-351.

Drugs and Lactation Database (LactMed) [Internet]. Bethesda (MD): National Library of Medicine (US); 2006; Available from http://www.ncbi.nlm.nih.gov/books/NBK501895/

Dutta A, Chakraborty A. Cinnamon in Anticancer Armamentarium: A Molecular Approach. *J Toxicol.* 2018:8978731.

Dybkowska E, Sadowska A, Rakowska R, Dębowska M, Świderski F, Świąder K. Assessing polyphenols content and antioxidant activity in coffee beans according to origin and the degree of roasting. *Rocz Panstw Zakl Hig.* 2017;68(4):347-353.

Ebrahimzadeh Attari V, Malek Mahdavi A, Javadivala Z, Mahluji S, Zununi Vahed S, Ostadrahimi A. A systematic review of the anti-obesity and weight lowering effect of ginger (*Zingiber officinale* Roscoe) and its mechanisms of action. *Phytother Res.* 2018;32(4):577-585.

Egras AM, Hamilton WR, Lenz TL, Monaghan MS. An evidence-based review of fat modifying supplemental weight loss products. *J Obes.* 2011;2011. pii: 297315.

El Rabey HA, Al-Seeni MN, Al-Ghamdi HB. Comparison between the Hypolipidemic Activity of Parsley and Carob in Hypercholesterolemic Male Rats. *Biomed Res Int.* 2017;2017:3098745. doi: 10.1155/2017/3098745.

Eyres L, Eyres MF, Chisholm A, Brown RC. Coconut oil consumption and cardiovascular risk factors in humans. *Nutr Rev.* 2016;74(4):267-80.

Fadare DA, Ajaiyeoba EO. Phytochemical and antimicrobial activities of the wild mango-*Irvingia gabonensis* extracts and fractions. *Afr J Med Med Sci.* 2008;37(2):119-24.

Fardet A, Chardigny JM. Plant-based foods as a source of lipotropes for human nutrition: a survey of *in vivo* studies. *Crit Rev Food Sci Nutr.* 2013;53(6):535-90.

Fassina P, Scherer Adami F, Terezinha Zani V, Kasper Machado IC, Garavaglia J, Quevedo Grave MT, Ramos R, Morelo Dal Bosco S. The effect of *Garcinia cambodgia* as coadjuvant in the weight loss process. *Nutr Hosp.* 2015;32(6):2400-8.:

Fernandes ES, Cerqueira AR, Soares AG, Costa SK. Capsaicin and Its Role in Chronic Diseases. *Adv Exp Med Biol.* 2016;929:91-125.

Fernando HA, Zibellini J, Harris RA, Seimon RV, Sainsbury A. Effect of Ramadan Fasting on Weight and Body Composition in Healthy Non-Athlete Adults: A Systematic Review and Meta-Analysis. *Nutrients.* 2019;11(2). pii: E478.

Ferrazzano GF, Cantile T, Alcidi B, Coda M, Ingenito A, Zarrelli A, Di Fabio G, Pollio A. Is *Stevia rebaudiana* Bertoni a Non Cariogenic Sweetener? A Review. *Molecules.* 2015;21(1):E38.

Flamm G, Glinsmann W, Kritchevsky D, Prosky L, Roberfroid M. Inulin and oligofructose as dietary fiber: a review of the evidence. *Crit Rev Food Sci Nutr.* 2001;41(5):353-62.

Flanagan J, Bily A, Rolland Y, Roller M. Lipolytic activity of Svetol®, a decaffeinated green coffee bean extract. *Phytother Res.* 2014;28(6):946-8.

Flatt JP. Conversion of carbohydrate to fat in adipose tissue: an energy-yielding and, therefore, self-limiting process. *J Lipid Res.* 1970;11(2):131-43.

Fotland TØ, Paulsen JE, Sanner T, Alexander J, Husøy T. Risk assessment of coumarin using the bench mark dose (BMD) approach: children in Norway which regularly eat oatmeal porridge with cinnamon may exceed the TDI for coumarin with several folds. *Food Chem Toxicol.* 2012;50(3-4):903-12.

Frost G, Sleeth ML, Sahuri-Arisoylu M, Lizarbe B, Cerdan S, Brody L, Anastasovska J, Ghourab S, Hankir M, Zhang S, Carling D, Swann JR, Gibson G, Viardot A, Morrison D, Louise Thomas E, Bell JD. The short-chain fatty acid acetate reduces appetite via a central homeostatic mechanism. *Nat Commun.* 2014;5:3611.

Furchner-Evanson A, Petrisko Y, Howarth L, Nemoseck T, Kern M. Type of snack influences satiety responses in adult women. *Appetite.* 2010;54(3):564-9.

Fushimi T, Sato Y. Effect of acetic acid feeding on the circadian changes in glycogen and metabolites of glucose and lipid in liver and skeletal muscle of rats. *Br J Nutr.* 2005;94(5):714-9.

Gambero A, Ribeiro ML. The positive effects of yerba maté (*Ilex paraguariensis*) in obesity. *Nutrients.* 2015;7(2):730-50.

Gamboa-Gómez CI, Rocha-Guzmán NE, Gallegos-Infante JA, Moreno-Jiménez MR, Vázquez-Cabral BD, González-Laredo RF. Plants with potential use on obesity and its complications. *EXCLI J.* 2015;14:809-31.

Gambon DL, Brand HS, Veerman EC. [Unhealthy weight loss. Erosion by apple cider vinegar]. *Ned Tijdschr Tandheelkd.* 2012;119(12):589-91.

Ganesan K, Habboush Y, Sultan S. Intermittent Fasting: The Choice for a Healthier Lifestyle. *Cureus.* 2018;10(7):e2947.

Gannon NP, Lambalot EL, Vaughan RA. The effects of capsaicin and capsaicinoid analogs on metabolic molecular targets in highly energetic tissues and cell types. *Biofactors.* 2016;42(3):229-46.

García-Montalvo IA, Méndez Díaz SY, Aguirre Guzmán N, Sánchez Medina MA, Matías Pérez D, Pérez Campos E. [Increasing consumption of dietary fiber complementary to the treatment of metabolic syndrome]. *Nutr Hosp.* 2018;35(3):582-7.

Gardner C. Non-nutritive sweeteners: evidence for benefit vs. risk. *Curr Opin Lipidol.* 2014;25(1):80-4.

Gbadegesin MA, Adegoke AM, Ewere EG, Odunola OA. Hepatoprotective and anticlastogenic effects of ethanol extract of *Irvingia gabonensis* (IG) leaves in sodium arsenite-induced toxicity in male Wistar rats. *Niger J Physiol Sci.* 2014;29(1):29-36.

Geliebter A, Astbury NM, Aviram-Friedman R, Yahav E, Hashim S. Skipping breakfast leads to weight loss but also elevated cholesterol compared with consuming daily breakfasts of oat porridge or frosted cornflakes in overweight individuals: a randomised controlled trial. *J Nutr Sci.* 2014;3:e56.

Genta S, Cabrera W, Habib N, Pons J, Carillo IM, Grau A, Sánchez S. Yacon syrup: beneficial effects on obesity and insulin resistance in humans. *Clin Nutr.* 2009;28(2):182-7.

Geuns JM. Stevioside. *Phytochemistry.* 2003;64(5):913-21.

Ghaben AL, Scherer PE. Adipogenesis and metabolic health. *Nat Rev Mol Cell Biol.* 2019;20(4):242-258.

Gilissen LJWJ, van der Meer IM, Smulders MJM. Why Oats Are Safe and Healthy for Celiac Disease Patients. *Med Sci* (Basel). 2016;4(4). pii: E21.

Giralt M, Villarroya F. White, brown, beige/brite: different adipose cells for different functions? *Endocrinology.* 2013;154(9):2992-3000.

Gomes da Silva MF, Dionísio AP, Ferreira Carioca AA, Silveira Adriano L, Pinto CO, Pinto de Abreu FA, Wurlitzer NJ, Araújo IM, Dos Santos Garruti D, Ferreira Pontes D. Yacon syrup: Food applications and impact on satiety in healthy volunteers. *Food Res Int.* 2017;100(Pt 1):460-7.

Greenway FL, Liu Z, Martin CK, Kai-yuan W, Nofziger J, Rood JC, Yu Y, Amen RJ. Safety and efficacy of NT, an herbal supplement, in treating human obesity. *Int J Obes* (Lond). 2006;30(12):1737-41.

Gregersen NT, Belza A, Jensen MG, Ritz C, Bitz C, Hels O, Frandsen E, Mela DJ, Astrup A. Acute effects of mustard, horseradish, black pepper and ginger on energy expenditure, appetite, ad libitum energy intake and energy balance in human subjects. *Br J Nutr.* 2013;109(3):556-63.

Guess ND, Dornhorst A, Oliver N, Bell JD, Thomas EL, Frost GS. A randomized controlled trial: the effect of inulin on weight management and ectopic fat in subjects with prediabetes. *Nutr Metab* (Lond). 2015;12:36.

Gulati S, Misra A, Pandey RM. Effects of 3 g of soluble fiber from oats on lipid levels of Asian Indians - a randomized controlled, parallel arm study. *Lipids Health Dis.* 2017;16(1):71.

Gupta Jain S, Puri S, Misra A, Gulati S, Mani K. Effect of oral cinnamon intervention on metabolic profile and body composition of Asian Indians with metabolic syndrome: a randomized double -blind control trial. *Lipids Health Dis.* 2017;16(1):113.

Hackman RM, Havel PJ, Schwartz HJ, Rutledge JC, Watnik MR, Noceti EM, Stohs SJ, Stern JS, Keen CL. Multinutrient supplement containing ephedra and caffeine causes weight loss and improves metabolic risk factors in obese women: a randomized controlled trial. *Int J Obes* (Lond). 2006;30(10):1545-56.

Haider N, Larose L. Harnessing adipogenesis to prevent obesity. *Adipocyte.* 2019:1-7.

Hajimonfarednejad M, Ostovar M, Raee MJ, Hashempur MH, Mayer JG, Heydari M. Cinnamon: A systematic review of adverse events. *Clin Nutr.* 2018; pii: S0261-5614(18)30125-0.

Han SF, Jiao J, Zhang W, Xu JY, Zhang W, Fu CL, Qin LQ. Lipolysis and thermogenesis in adipose tissues as new potential mechanisms for metabolic benefits of dietary fiber. *Nutrition.* 2017;33:118-24.

Haque MA, Jantan I. Recent Updates on the Phytochemistry, Pharmacological, and Toxicological Activities of *Zingiber zerumbet* (L.) Roscoe ex Sm. *Curr Pharm Biotechnol.* 2017;18(9):696-720.

Hariri M, Ghiasvand R. Cinnamon and Chronic Diseases. *Adv Exp Med Biol.* 2016;929:1-24.

Harrold JA, Hughes GM, O'Shiel K, Quinn E, Boyland EJ, Williams NJ, Halford JC. Acute effects of a herb extract formulation and inulin fibre on appetite, energy intake and food choice. *Appetite.* 2013;62:84-90.

Hasani-Ranjbar S, Nayebi N, Larijani B, Abdollahi M. A systematic review of the efficacy and safety of herbal medicines used in the treatment of obesity. *World J Gastroenterol.* 2009;15(25):3073-85.

Hayamizu K, Tomi H, Kaneko I, Shen M, Soni MG, Yoshino G. Effects of Garcinia cambogia extract on serum sex hormones in overweight subjects. *Fitoterapia.* 2008;79(4):255-61.

Haylett WL, Ferris WF. Adipocyte-progenitor cell communication that influences adipogenesis. *Cell Mol Life Sci.* 2019; 77(1):115-28.

He X, Fang J, Ruan Y, Wang X, Sun Y, Wu N, Zhao Z, Chang Y, Ning N, Guo H, Huang L. Structures, bioactivities and future prospective of polysaccharides from *Morus alba* (white mulberry): A review. *Food Chem.* 2018;245:899-910.

Hess JR, Birkett AM, Thomas W, Slavin JL. Effects of short-chain fructooligosaccharides on satiety responses in healthy men and women. *Appetite.* 2011;56(1):128-34.

Heymsfield SB, Allison DB, Vasselli JR, Pietrobelli A, Greenfield D, Nunez C Garcinia cambogia (hydroxycitric acid) as a potential antiobesity agent: a randomized controlled trial. *JAMA.* 1998;280(18):1596-600.

Hill LL, Woodruff LH, Foote JC, Barreto-Alcoba M. Esophageal injury by apple cider vinegar tablets and subsequent evaluation of products. *J Am Diet Assoc.* 2005;105(7):1141-4.

Ho HVT, Jovanovski E, Zurbau A, Blanco Mejia S, Sievenpiper JL, Au-Yeung F, Jenkins AL, Duvnjak L, Leiter L, Vuksan V. A systematic review and meta-analysis of randomized controlled trials of the effect of konjac glucomannan, a viscous soluble fiber, on LDL cholesterol and the new lipid targets non-HDL cholesterol and apolipoprotein B. *Am J Clin Nutr.* 2017;105(5):1239-1247.

Hochkogler CM, Hoi JK, Lieder B, Müller N, Hans J, Widder S, Ley JP, Somoza V. Cinnamyl Isobutyrate Decreases Plasma Glucose Levels and Total Energy Intake from a Standardized Breakfast: A Randomized, Crossover Intervention. *Mol Nutr Food Res.* 2018;62(17):e1701038.

Hosni AA, Abdel-Moneim AA, Abdel-Reheim ES, Mohamed SM, Helmy H. Cinnamaldehyde potentially attenuates gestational hyperglycemia in rats through modulation of PPARγ, proinflammatory cytokines and oxidative stress. *Biomed Pharmacother*. 2017;88:52-60.

Howarth L, Petrisko Y, Furchner-Evanson A, Nemoseck T, Kern M. Snack selection influences nutrient intake, triglycerides, and bowel habits of adult women: a pilot study. *J Am Diet Assoc*. 2010;110(9):1322-7.

Hu J, Webster D, Cao J, Shao A. The safety of green tea and green tea extract consumption in adults - Results of a systematic review. *Regul Toxicol Pharmacol*. 2018;95:412-33.

Huang J, Wang Y, Xie Z, Zhou Y, Zhang Y, Wan X. The anti-obesity effects of green tea in human intervention and basic molecular studies. *Eur J Clin Nutr*. 2014;68(10):1075-87.

Igho O, Shao K, Rachel P, Barbara W, Edzard E. "The Use of Garcinia Extract Hydroxycitric Acid as a Weight loss Supplement: A Systematic Review and Meta-Analysis of Randomised Clinical Trials. *J Obes*. 2011 (622): 849.

Igwe EO, Charlton KE. A Systematic Review on the Health Effects of Plums (*Prunus domestica* and *Prunus salicina*). *Phytother Res*. 2016;30(5):701-31.

Irandoost P, Ebrahimi-Mameghani M, Pirouzpanah S. Does grape seed oil improve inflammation and insulin resistance in overweight or obese women? *Int J Food Sci Nutr*. 2013;64(6):706-10.

Isaac-Renton M, Li MK, Parsons LM. Cinnamon spice and everything not nice: many features of intraoral allergy to cinnamic aldehyde. *Dermatitis*. 2015;26(3):116-21.

Islam MT, Tabrez S, Jabir NR, Ali M, Kamal MA, da Silva Araujo L, De Oliveira Santos JV, Da Mata AMOF, De Aguiar RPS, de Carvalho Melo Cavalcante AA. An Insight into the Therapeutic Potential of Major Coffee Components. *Curr Drug Metab*. 2018;19(6):544-556.

Jamous RM, Abu-Zaitoun SY, Akkawi RJ, Ali-Shtayeh MS. Antiobesity and Antioxidant Potentials of Selected Palestinian Medicinal Plants. *Evid Based Complement Alternat Med*. 2018;2018:8426752.

Jamous RM, Abu-Zaitoun SY, Akkawi RJ, Ali-Shtayeh MS. Antiobesity and antioxidant potentials of selected palestinian medicinal plants. *Evid*

Based Complement Alternat Med. 2018;8426752. doi: 10.1155/2018/8426752.

Jane M, McKay J, Pal S. Effects of daily consumption of psyllium, oat bran and polyGlycopleX on obesity-related disease risk factors: A critical review. *Nutrition.* 2019;57:84-91.

Janssens PL, Hursel R, Westerterp-Plantenga MS. Nutraceuticals for body-weight management: The role of green tea catechins. *Physiol Behav.* 2016;162:83-7.

Javadi L, Khoshbaten M, Safaiyan A, Ghavami M, Abbasi MM, Gargari BP. Pro- and prebiotic effects on oxidative stress and inflammatory markers in non-alcoholic fatty liver disease. *Asia Pac J Clin Nutr.* 2018;27(5):1031-1039.

Jena BS, Jayaprakasha GK, Singh RP, Sakariah KK. Chemistry and biochemistry of (-)-hydroxycitric acid from Garcinia. *J Agric Food Chem.* 2002;50(1):10-22.

Jiang J, Emont MP, Jun H, Qiao X, Liao J, Kim DI, Wu J. Cinnamaldehyde induces fat cell-autonomous thermogenesis and metabolic reprogramming. *Metabolism.* 2017;77:58-64.

Johnston CS, Buller AJ. Vinegar and peanut products as complementary foods to reduce postprandial glycemia. *J Am Diet Assoc.* 2005;105(12):1939-42.

Johnston CS. Strategies for healthy weight loss: from vitamin C to the glycemic response. *J Am Coll Nutr.* 2005;24(3):158-65.

Jongberg S, Racanicci AMC, Skibsted LH. Mate extract is superior to green tea extract in the protection against chicken meat protein thiol oxidation. *Food Chem.* 2019;300:125134.

Kalantari K, Moniri M, Boroumand Moghaddam A, Abdul Rahim R, Bin Ariff A, Izadiyan Z, Mohamad R. A Review of the Biomedical Applications of Zerumbone and the Techniques for Its Extraction from Ginger Rhizomes. *Molecules.* 2017;22(10). pii: E1645.

Karak T, Kutu FR, Nath JR, Sonar I, Paul RK, Boruah RK, Sanyal S, Sabhapondit S, Dutta AK. Micronutrients (B, Co, Cu, Fe, Mn, Mo, and Zn) content in made tea (*Camellia sinensis* L.) and tea infusion with health prospect: A critical review. *Crit Rev Food Sci Nutr.* 2017;57(14):2996-3034.

Karri S, Sharma S, Hatware K, Patil K. Natural anti-obesity agents and their therapeutic role in management of obesity: A future trend perspective. *Biomed Pharmacother.* 2019;110:224-38.

Kawabata F, Inoue N, Yazawa S, Kawada T, Inoue K, Fushiki T. Effects of CH-19 sweet, a non-pungent cultivar of red pepper, in decreasing the body weight and suppressing body fat accumulation by sympathetic nerve activation in humans. *Biosci Biotechnol Biochem.* 2006; 70(12):2824-35.

Kawatra P, Rajagopalan R. Cinnamon: Mystic powers of a minute ingredient. *Pharmacognosy Res.* 2015;7(Suppl 1):S1-6.

Keithley J, Swanson B. Glucomannan and obesity: a critical review. *Altern Ther Health Med.* 2005;11(6):30-4.

Khatib, S., J. Vaya, Chapter 17 - Fig, Carob, Pistachio, and Health. In: *Bioactive Foods in Promoting Health* (R.R. Watson and V.R. Preedy eds.), Academic Press, New York-London, 2010;245-263, ISBN 9780123746283, doi.org/10.1016/B978-0-12-374628-3.00017-7.

Kim H, Cho KW, Jeong J, Park K, Ryu Y, Moyo KM, Kim HK, Go GW. Red Pepper (*Capsicum annuum* L.) Seed Extract Decreased Hepatic Gluconeogenesis and Increased Muscle Glucose Uptake In Vitro. *J Med Food.* 2018;21(7):665-671.

Kim H, Kim DH, Seo KH, Chon JW, Nah SY, Bartley GE, Arvik T, Lipson R, Yokoyama W. Modulation of the intestinal microbiota is associated with lower plasma cholesterol and weight gain in hamsters fed chardonnay grape seed flour. *J Agric Food Chem.* 2015;63(5):1460-7.

Kim SY, Oh MR, Kim MG, Chae HJ, Chae SW. Anti-obesity effects of Yerba Mate (*Ilex paraguariensis*): a randomized, double-blind, placebo-controlled clinical trial. *BMC Complement Altern Med.* 2015;15:338.

Kim Y, Talcott ST. Tea creaming in nonfermented teas from Camellia sinensis and Ilex vomitoria. *J Agric Food Chem.* 2012;60(47):11793-9.

Kondo S, Tayama K, Tsukamoto Y, Ikeda K, Yamori Y. Antihypertensive effects of acetic acid and vinegar on spontaneously hypertensive rats. *Biosci Biotechnol Biochem.* 2001;65(12):2690-4.

Kondo T, Kishi M, Fushimi T, Ugajin S, Kaga T. Vinegar intake reduces body weight, body fat mass, and serum triglyceride levels in obese Japanese subjects. *Biosci Biotechnol Biochem.* 2009;73(8):1837-43.

Korczak R, Slavin JL. Fructooligosaccharides and appetite. *Curr Opin Clin Nutr Metab Care.* 2018;21(5):377-380.

Kothadia JP, Kaminski M, Samant H, Olivera-Martinez M. Hepatotoxicity Associated with Use of the Weight Loss Supplement Garcinia cambogia: A Case Report and Review of the Literature. *Case Reports Hepatol.* 2018;2018:6483605.

Kothari SC, Shivarudraiah P, Venkataramaiah SB, Gavara S, Soni MG. Subchronic toxicity and mutagenicity/genotoxicity studies of Irvingia gabonensis extract (IGOB131). *Food Chem Toxicol.* 2012;50(5):1468-79.

Kralik R, Roubalova M, Lenovsky L, Tuska T, Kralj-Vuksic S. Taanit bechorim (Fast on the first-born) in rabbinic judaism. *XLingue* 2018;11(2):17-23.

Kristensen M, Damgaard TW, Sørensen AD, Raben A, Lindeløv TS, Thomsen AD, Bjergegaard C, Sørensen H, Astrup A, Tetens I. Whole flaxseeds but not sunflower seeds in rye bread reduce apparent digestibility of fat in healthy volunteers. *Eur J Clin Nutr.* 2008;62(8):961-7.

Kudiganti V, Kodur RR, Kodur SR, Halemane M, Deep DK. Efficacy and tolerability of Meratrim for weight management: a randomized, double-blind, placebo-controlled study in healthy overweight human subjects. *Lipids Health Dis.* 2016;15(1):136.

Lachman J, Fernández EC, Orsák M. Yacon [*Smallanthus sonchifolia* (Poepp. et Endl.) H. Robinson] chemical composition and use – a review. *Plant Soil Environ.* 2003;49(6): 283–90.

Lakkab I, Hajaji HE, Lachkar N, Bali BE, Lachkar M, Ciobica A. Phytochemistry, bioactivity: suggestion of *Ceratonia siliqua* L. as neurodegenerative disease therapy. *J Complement Integr Med.* 2018;15(4). pii:/j/jcim.2018.15.issue-4/jcim-2018-0013/jcim-2018-0013.xml. doi:10.1515/jcim-2018-0013.

Landor M, Benami A, Segev N, Loberant B. Efficacy and acceptance of a commercial *Hoodia parviflora* product for support of appetite and weight control in a consumer trial. *J Med Food.* 2015;18(2):250-8.

Lee YM, Yoon Y, Yoon H, Park HM, Song S, Yeum KJ. Dietary Anthocyanins against Obesity and Inflammation. *Nutrients.* 2017;9(10). pii: E1089.

Lemus-Mondaca R, Vega-Gálvez A, Zura-Bravo L, Ah-Hen K. Stevia rebaudiana Bertoni, source of a high-potency natural sweetener: A comprehensive review on the biochemical, nutritional and functional aspects. *Food Chem.* 2012;132(3):1121-1132.

Lhotta K, Höfle G, Gasser R, Finkenstedt G. Hypokalemia, hyperreninemia and osteoporosis in a patient ingesting large amounts of cider vinegar. *Nephron.* 1998;80(2):242-3.

Li AN, Chen JJ, Li QQ, Zeng GY, Chen QY, Chen JL, Liao ZM, Jin P, Wang KS, Yang ZC. Alpha-glucosidase inhibitor 1-Deoxynojirimycin promotes beige remodeling of 3T3-L1 preadipocytes via activating AMPK. *Biochem Biophys Res Commun.* 2019;509(4):1001-1007.

Li X, Cai X, Ma X, Jing L, Gu J, Bao L, Li J, Xu M, Zhang Z, Li Y. Short- and long-term effects of wholegrain oat intake on weight management and glucolipid metabolism in overweight type-2 diabetics: a randomized control trial. *Nutrients.* 2016;8(9). pii: E549.

Li Y, Wang C, Huai Q, Guo F, Liu L, Feng R, Sun C. Effects of tea or tea extract on metabolic profiles in patients with type 2 diabetes mellitus: a meta-analysis of ten randomized controlled trials. *Diabetes Metab Res Rev.* 2016;32(1):2-10.

Liljeberg H, Björck I. Delayed gastric emptying rate may explain improved glycaemia in healthy subjects to a starchy meal with added vinegar. *Eur J Clin Nutr.* 1998;52(5):368-71

Lim SH, Choi CI. Pharmacological Properties of *Morus nigra* L. (Black Mulberry) as A Promising Nutraceutical Resource. *Nutrients.* 2019;11(2). pii: E437.

Lin Z, Zhang B, Liu X, Jin R, Zhu W. Effects of chicory inulin on serum metabolites of uric acid, lipids, glucose, and abdominal fat deposition in quails induced by purine-rich diets. *J Med Food.* 2014;17(11):1214-21.

Liu F, Prabhakar M, Ju J, Long H, Zhou HW. Effect of inulin-type fructans on blood lipid profile and glucose level: a systematic review and meta-analysis of randomized controlled trials. *Eur J Clin Nutr.* 2017;71(1):9-20.

Liu Y, Cotillard A, Vatier C, Bastard JP, Fellahi S, Stévant M, Allatif O, Langlois C, Bieuvelet S, Brochot A, Guilbot A, Clément K, Rizkalla SW. A Dietary supplement containing cinnamon, chromium and carnosine decreases fasting plasma glucose and increases lean mass in overweight or obese pre-diabetic subjects: a randomized, placebo-controlled trial. *PLoS One.* 2015;10(9):e0138646.

Lobb A. Hepatoxicity associated with weight-loss supplements: a case for better post-marketing surveillance. *World J Gastroenterol.* 2009;15(14):1786-7.

Lohner S, Toews I, Meerpohl JJ. Health outcomes of non-nutritive sweeteners: analysis of the research landscape. *Nutr J.* 2017;16(1):55.

Lopes SM, Krausová G, Carneiro JW, Gonçalves JE, Gonçalves RA, de Oliveira AJ. A new natural source for obtainment of inulin and fructo-oligosaccharides from industrial waste of Stevia rebaudiana Bertoni. *Food Chem.* 2017;225:154-61.

Lu M, Cao Y, Xiao J, Song M, Ho CT. Molecular mechanisms of the anti-obesity effect of bioactive ingredients in common spices: a review. *Food Funct.* 2018;9(9):4569-81.

Lüde S, Vecchio S, Sinno-Tellier S, Dopter A, Mustonen H, Vucinic S, Jonsson B, Müller D, Veras Gimenez Fruchtengarten L, Hruby K, De Souza Nascimento E, Di Lorenzo C, Restani P, Kupferschmidt H, Ceschi A. Adverse effects of plant food supplements and plants consumed as food: results from the poisons centres-based PlantLIBRA study. *Phytother Res.* 2016;30(6):988-96.

Ludwig IA, Clifford MN, Lean ME, Ashihara H, Crozier A. Coffee: biochemistry and potential impact on health. *Food Funct.* 2014;5(8):1695-717.

Ludy MJ, Mattes RD. The effects of hedonically acceptable red pepper doses on thermogenesis and appetite. *Physiol Behav.* 2011;102(3-4):251-8.

Luís Â, Domingues F, Pereira L. Metabolic changes after licorice consumption: A systematic review with meta-analysis and trial sequential analysis of clinical trials. *Phytomedicine.* 2018;39:17-24.

Luo K, Wang X, Zhang G. The anti-obesity effect of starch in a whole grain-like structural form. Food Funct. 2018;9(7):3755-3763.

Lynch B, Lau A, Baldwin N, Bauter MR, Marone PA. Subchronic and reproductive toxicity of whole dried *Hoodia parviflora* aerial parts in the rat. *Food Chem Toxicol.* 2013;56:313-24.

MacLean DB, Luo LG. Increased ATP content/production in the hypothalamus may be a signal for energy-sensing of satiety: studies of the anorectic mechanism of a plant steroidal glycoside. *Brain Res.* 2004;1020(1-2):1-11.

Madgula VL, Ashfaq MK, Wang YH, Avula B, Khan IA, Walker LA, Khan SI. Bioavailability, pharmacokinetics, and tissue distribution of the oxypregnane steroidal glycoside P57AS3 (P57) from *Hoodia gordonii* in mouse model. *Planta Med.* 2010;76(14):1582-6.

Maharlouei N, Tabrizi R, Lankarani KB, Rezaianzadeh A, Akbari M, Kolahdooz F, Rahimi M, Keneshlou F, Asemi Z. The effects of ginger intake on weight loss andmetabolic profiles among overweight and obese subjects: A systematic review and meta-analysis of randomized controlled trials. *Crit Rev Food Sci Nutr.* 2019;59(11):1753-66.

Mahboubi M. *Morus alba* (mulberry), a natural potent compound in management of obesity. *Pharmacol Res.* 2019;104341.

Mahmoudi M, Charradi K, Limam F, Aouani E. Grape seed and skin extract as an adjunct to xenical therapy reduces obesity, brain lipotoxicity and oxidative stress in high fat diet fed rats. *Obes Res Clin Pract.* 2018;12(1S1):115-26.

Maia-Landim A, Ramírez JM, Lancho C, Poblador MS, Lancho JL. Long-term effects of *Garcinia cambogia*/Glucomannan on weight loss in people with obesity, PLIN4, FTO and Trp64Arg polymorphisms. *BMC Complement Altern Med.* 2018;18(1):26.

Maierean SM, Serban MC, Sahebkar A, Ursoniu S, Serban A, Penson P, Banach M; Lipid and Blood Pressure Meta-analysis Collaboration (LBPMC) Group. The effects of cinnamon supplementation on blood lipid concentrations: A systematic review and meta-analysis. *J Clin Lipidol*. 2017;11(6):1393-1406.

Majzoobi M, Mohammadi M, Mesbahi G, Farahnaky A. Feasibility study of sucrose and fat replacement using inulin and rebaudioside A in cake formulations. *J Texture Stud*. 2018;49(5):468-475.

Mallika J, Shyamala CSD. In vitro and In vivo evaluation of free radical scavenging potential of *Cissus quadrangularis*. *Afri J Biomed Res*. 2005, 8: 95-99.

Malongane F, McGaw LJ, Mudau FN. The synergistic potential of various teas, herbs and therapeutic drugs in health improvement: a review. *J Sci Food Agric*. 2017;97(14):4679-89.

Mansour MS, Ni YM, Roberts AL, Kelleman M, Roychoudhury A, St-Onge MP. Ginger consumption enhances the thermic effect of food and promotes feelings of satiety without affecting metabolic and hormonal parameters in overweight men: a pilot study. *Metabolism*. 2012;61(10):1347-52.

Marcinek K, Krejpcio Z. Chia seeds (Salvia hispanica): health promoting properties and therapeutic applications – a review. *Rocz Panstw Zakl Hig*. 2017;68(2):123-129.

Markey O, McClean CM, Medlow P, Davison GW, Trinick TR, Duly E, Shafat A. Effect of cinnamon on gastric emptying, arterial stiffness, postprandial lipemia, glycemia, and appetite responses to high-fat breakfast. *Cardiovasc Diabetol*. 2011;10:78.

Martinchik AN, Baturin AK, Zubtsov VV, Molofeev VIu. [Nutritional value and functional properties of flaxseed]. *Vopr Pitan*. 2012;81(3):4-10.

Martínez-Rodríguez R, Navarro-Alarcón M, Rodríguez-Martínez C, Fonollá-Joya J.[Effects on the lipid profile in humans of a polyphenol-rich carob (*Ceratonia siliqua* L.) extract in a dairy matrix like a functional food; a pilot study]. *Nutr Hosp*. 2013;28(6):2107-14. doi: 10.3305/nutr hosp.v28in06.6952.

Martínez-Villaluenga C, Peñas E, Rico D, Martin-Diana AB, Portillo MP, Macarulla MT, de Luis DA, Miranda J. Potential Usefulness of a Wakame/Carob Functional Snack for the Treatment of Several Aspects of Metabolic Syndrome: From *In Vitro* to *In Vivo* Studies. *Mar Drugs.* 2018;16(12). pii: E512. doi:10.3390/md16120512.

Matesanz N, Nikolic I, Leiva M, Pulgarín-Alfaro M, Santamans AM, Bernardo E, Mora A, Herrera-Melle L, Rodríguez E, Beiroa D, Caballero A, Martín-García E, Acín-Pérez R, Hernández-Cosido L, Leiva-Vega L, Torres JL, Centeno F, Nebreda AR, Enríquez JA, Nogueiras R, Marcos M, Sabio G. p38α blocks brown adipose tissue thermogenesis through p38δ inhibition. *PLoS Biol.* 2018;16(7):e2004455.

Mattes RD, Bormann L. Effects of (-)-hydroxycitric acid on appetitive variables. *Physiol Behav.* 2000;71(1-2):87-94.

Maufrais C, Sarafian D, Dulloo A, Montani JP. Cardiovascular and Metabolic Responses to the Ingestion of Caffeinated Herbal Tea: Drink It Hot or Cold? *Front Physiol.* 2018;9:315.

Mazzanti G, Di Sotto A, Vitalone A. Hepatotoxicity of green tea: an update. *Arch Toxicol.* 2015;89(8):1175-91.

Medagama AB. The glycaemic outcomes of Cinnamon, a review of the experimental evidence and clinical trials. *Nutr J.* 2015;14:108.

Méndez-Del Villar M, González-Ortiz M, Martínez-Abundis E, Pérez-Rubio KG, Cortez-Navarrete M. Effect of Irvingia gabonensis on Metabolic Syndrome, Insulin Sensitivity, and Insulin Secretion. *J Med Food.* 2018;21(6):568-574.

Mensink MA, Frijlink HW, van der Voort Maarschalk K, Hinrichs WL. Inulin, a flexible oligosaccharide I: Review of its physicochemical characteristics. *Carbohydr Polym.* 2015;130:405-19.

Messina D, Soto C, Méndez A, Corte C, Kemnitz M, Avena V, Del Balzo D, Pérez Elizalde R. [Lipid - lowering effect of mate tea intake in dyslipidemic subjects]. *Nutr Hosp.* 2015;31(5):2131-9.

Metwally FM, Rashad H, Mahmoud AA. Morus alba L. Diminishes visceral adiposity, insulin resistance, behavioral alterations via regulation of gene expression of leptin, resistin and adiponectin in rats fed a high-cholesterol diet. *Physiol Behav.* 2019;201:1-11.

Mielgo-Ayuso J, Barrenechea L, Alcorta P, Larrarte E, Margareto J, Labayen I. Effects of dietary supplementation with epigallocatechin-3-

gallate on weight loss, energy homeostasis, cardiometabolic risk factors and liver function in obese women: randomised, double-blind, placebo-controlled clinical trial. *Br J Nutr*. 2014;111(7):1263-71.

Miglio C, Peluso I, Raguzzini A, Villaño DV, Cesqui E, Catasta G, Toti E, Serafini M. Fruit juice drinks prevent endogenous antioxidant response to high-fat meal ingestion. *Br J Nutr*. 2014;111(2):294-300.

Mishra G, Srivastava S, Nagori BP. Pharmacological and Therapeutic Activity of *Cissus quadrangularis*: An Overview. *Int J PharmTech Res*. 2010; 2:1298-1310.

Mohamed GA, Ibrahim SRM, Elkhayat ES, El Dine RS. Natural anti-obesity agents. *Bull Fac Pharmacy*, Cairo University 2014; 52:269-284.

Mohd-Radzman NH, Ismail WI, Adam Z, Jaapar SS, Adam A. Potential Roles of Stevia rebaudiana Bertoni in Abrogating Insulin Resistance and Diabetes: A Review. *Evid Based Complement Alternat Med*. 2013;2013:718049.

Mollazadeh H, Hosseinzadeh H. Cinnamon effects on metabolic syndrome: a review based on its mechanisms. *Iran J Basic Med Sci*. 2016;19(12):1258-1270.

Momtazi-Borojeni AA, Esmaeili SA, Abdollahi E, Sahebkar A. A Review on the Pharmacology and Toxicology of Steviol Glycosides Extracted from *Stevia rebaudiana*. *Curr Pharm Des*. 2017;23(11):1616-22.

Monzani A, Ricotti R, Caputo M, Solito A, Archero F, Bellone S, Prodam F. A Systematic Review of the Association of Skipping Breakfast with Weight and Cardiometabolic Risk Factors in Children and Adolescents. What Should We Better Investigate in the Future? *Nutrients*. 2019;11(2). pii: E387.

Morabbi Najafabad A, Jamei R. Free radical scavenging capacity and antioxidant activity of methanolic and ethanolic extracts of plum (*Prunus domestica* L.) in both fresh and dried samples. *Avicenna J Phytomed*. 2014;4(5):343-53.

Mosqueda-Solís A, Sánchez J, Portillo MP, Palou A, Picó C. Combination of Capsaicin and Hesperidin Reduces the Effectiveness of Each Compound To Decrease the Adipocyte Size and To Induce Browning

Features in Adipose Tissue of Western Diet Fed Rats. *J Agric Food Chem*. 2018;66(37):9679-89.

Namdar H, Emaratkar E, Hadavand MB. Persian Traditional Medicine and Ocular Health. *Med Hypothesis Discov Innov Ophthalmol*. 2015 Winter; 4(4):162-166.

Nangue TJ, Womeni HM, Mbiapo FT, Fanni J, Michel L. *Irvingia gabonensis* fat: nutritional properties and effect of increasing amounts on the growth and lipid metabolism of young rats wistar sp. *Lipids Health Dis*. 2011;10:43.

Nazıroğlu M, Güler M, Özgül C, Saydam G, Küçükayaz M, Sözbir E. Apple cider vinegar modulates serum lipid profile, erythrocyte, kidney, and liver membrane oxidative stress in ovariectomized mice fed high cholesterol. *J Membr Biol*. 2014;247(8):667-73.

Neto JGO, Bento-Bernardes T, Pazos-Moura CC, Oliveira KJ. Maternal cinnamon intake during lactation led to visceral obesity and hepatic metabolic dysfunction in the adult male offspring. *Endocrine*. 2019; 63(3):520-30.

Ngondi JL, Etoundi BC, Nyangono CB, Mbofung CM, Oben JE. IGOB131, a novel seed extract of the West African plant *Irvingia gabonensis*, significantly reduces body weight and improves metabolic parameters in overweight humans in a randomized double-blind placebo-controlled investigation. *Lipids Health Dis*. 2009;8:7.

Ngondi JL, Oben JE, Minka SR. The effect of *Irvingia gabonensis* seeds on body weight and blood lipids of obese subjects in Cameroon. *Lipids Health Dis*. 2005;4:12.

Nieman DC, Cayea EJ, Austin MD, Henson DA, McAnulty SR, Jin F. Chia seed does not promote weight loss or alter disease risk factors in overweight adults. *Nutr Res*. 2009;29(6):414-8.

Noratto G, Martino HS, Simbo S, Byrne D, Mertens-Talcott SU. Consumption of polyphenol-rich peach and plum juice prevents risk factors for obesity-related metabolic disorders and cardiovascular disease in Zucker rats. *J Nutr Biochem*. 2015;26(6):633-41.

Noratto GD, Garcia-Mazcorro JF, Markel M, Martino HS, Minamoto Y, Steiner JM, Byrne D, Suchodolski JS, Mertens-Talcott SU.

Carbohydrate-Free Peach (*Prunus persica*) and Plum (*Prunus salicina*) [corrected] Juice affects fecal microbial ecology in an obese animal model. *PLoS One.* 2014;9(7):e101723.

Nowak A, Czkwianianc E. A contemporary approach to body mass regulation mechanisms. *Prz Gastroenterol.* 2016;11(2):73-7.

Nowak-Węgrzyn A, Jarocka-Cyrta E, Moschione Castro A. Food Protein-Induced Enterocolitis Syndrome. *J Investig Allergol Clin Immunol.* 2017;27(1):1-18.

Nweze NE, Ogidi A, Ngongeh LA. Anthelmintic potential of three plants used in Nigerian ethnoveterinary medicine. *Pharm Biol.* 2013;51(3):311-5.

O'Connor S, Chouinard-Castonguay S, Gagnon C, Rudkowska I. Prebiotics in the management of components of the metabolic syndrome. *Maturitas.* 2017;104:11-18.

O'Connor S, Chouinard-Castonguay S, Gagnon C, Rudkowska I. Prebiotics in the management of components of the metabolic syndrome. *Maturitas.* 2017;104:11-18.

Oben J, Kuate D, Agbor G, Momo C, Talla X. The use of a *Cissus quadrangularis* formulation in the management of weight loss and metabolic syndrome. *Lipids Health Dis.* 2006;5:24.

Oben JE, Ngondi JL, Blum K. Inhibition of *Irvingia gabonensis* seed extract (OB131) on adipogenesis as mediated via down regulation of the PPAR gamma and leptin genes and up-regulation of the adiponectin gene. *Lipids Health Dis.* 2008;7:44.

Oben JE, Ngondi JL, Momo CN, Agbor GA, Sobgui CS. The use of a *Cissus quadrangularis/Irvingia gabonensis* combination in the management of weight loss: a double-blind placebo-controlled study. *Lipids Health Dis.* 2008;7:12.

Odžaković B, Džinić N, Kukrić Z, Grujić S. Effect of roasting degree on the antioxidant activity of different Arabica coffee quality classes. *Acta Sci Pol Technol Aliment.* 2016;15(4):409-417.

Ojo OA, Ajiboye BO, Oyinloye BE, Ojo AB, Olarewaju OI. Protective effect of *Irvingia gabonensis* stem bark extract on cadmium-induced nephrotoxicity in rats. *Interdiscip Toxicol.* 2014;7(4):208-14.

Ojo OA, Ojo AB, Ajiboye BO, Oyinloye BE, Akinyemi AJ, Okesola MA, Boligon AA, de Campos MMA. Chromatographic fingerprint analysis, antioxidant properties, and inhibition of cholinergic enzymes (acetylcholinesterase and butyrylcholinesterase) of phenolic extracts from *Irvingia gabonensis* (Aubry-Lecomte ex O'Rorke) Baill bark. *J Basic Clin Physiol Pharmacol*. 2018;29(2):217-24.

Ojulari OV, Lee SG, Nam JO. Beneficial Effects of Natural Bioactive Compounds from *Hibiscus sabdariffa* L. on Obesity. *Molecules*. 2019;24(1). pii: E210.

Okolo CO, Johnson PB, Abdurahman EM, Abdu-Aguye I, Hussaini IM. Analgesic effect of *Irvingia gabonensis* stem bark extract. *J Ethnopharmacol*. 1995;45(2):125-9.

Oliveira-de-Lira L, Santos EMC, de Souza RF, Matos RJB, Silva MCD, Oliveira LDS, Nascimento TGD, Schemly PALS, Souza SL. Supplementation-Dependent Effects of Vegetable Oils with Varying Fatty Acid Compositions on Anthropometric and Biochemical Parameters in Obese Women. *Nutrients*. 2018;10(7). pii: E932.

Oliveira-de-Lira L, Santos EMC, de Souza RF, Matos RJB, Silva MCD, Oliveira LDS, Nascimento TGD, Schemly PALS, Souza SL. Supplementation-dependent effects of vegetable oils with varying fatty acid compositions on anthropometric and biochemical parameters in obese women. *Nutrients*. 2018;10(7). pii: E932.

Omoruyi F, Adamson I. Digestive and hepatic enzymes in streptozotocin-induced diabetic rats fed supplements of dikanut (*Irvingia gabonensis*) and cellulose. *Ann Nutr Metab*. 1993;37(1):14-23.

Onakpoya I, Davies L, Posadzki P, Ernst E. The efficacy of *Irvingia gabonensis* supplementation in the management of overweight and obesity: a systematic review of randomized controlled trials. *J Diet Suppl*. 2013;10(1):29-38.

Onakpoya I, Hung SK, Perry R, Wider B, Ernst E. The Use of Garcinia Extract (Hydroxycitric Acid) as a Weight loss Supplement: A Systematic Review and Meta-Analysis of Randomised Clinical Trials. *J Obes*. 2011;2011:509038.

Onakpoya I, Posadzki P, Ernst E. The efficacy of glucomannan supplementation in overweight and obesity: a systematic review and meta-analysis of randomized clinical trials. *J Am Coll Nutr.* 2014;33(1):70-8.

Onakpoya I, Terry R, Ernst E. The use of green coffee extract as a weight loss supplement: a systematic review and meta-analysis of randomised clinical trials. *Gastroenterol Res Pract.* 2011;2011. pii: 382852.

Opala T, Rzymski P, Pischel I, Wilczak M, Wozniak J. Efficacy of 12 weeks supplementation of a botanical extract-based weight loss formula on body weight, body composition and blood chemistry in healthy, overweight subjects—a randomised double-blind placebo-controlled clinical trial. *Eur J Med Res.* 2006;11(8):343-50.

Oussaada SM, van Galen KA, Cooiman MI, Kleinendorst L, Hazebroek EJ, van Haelst MM, Ter Horst KW, Serlie MJ. The pathogenesis of obesity. *Metabolism.* 2019;92:26-36.

Oz HS. Chronic inflammatory diseases and green tea polyphenols. *Nutrients.* 2017;9(6). pii: E561.

Pan H, Gao Y, Tu Y. Mechanisms of Body Weight Reduction by Black Tea Polyphenols. *Molecules.* 2016;21(12). pii: E1659.

Pan J, Jiang Y, Lv Y, Li M, Zhang S, Liu J, Zhu Y, Zhang H. Comparison of the main compounds in Fuding white tea infusions from various tea types. *Food Sci Biotechnol.* 2018;27(5):1311-8.

Pan MH, Tung YC, Yang G, Li S, Ho CT. Molecular mechanisms of the anti-obesity effect of bioactive compounds in tea and coffee. *Food Funct.* 2016;7(11):4481-4491.

Paoli A, Tinsley G, Bianco A, Moro T. The Influence of Meal Frequency and Timing on Health in Humans: The Role of Fasting. *Nutrients.* 2019;11(4). pii: E719.

Parikh M, Netticadan T, Pierce GN. Flaxseed: its bioactive components and their cardiovascular benefits. *Am J Physiol Heart Circ Physiol.* 2018;314(2):H146-H159.

Parker J, Schellenberger AN, Roe AL, Oketch-Rabah H, Calderón AI. Therapeutic Perspectives on Chia Seed and Its Oil: A Review. *Planta Med.* 2018;84(9-10):606-612.

Peluso I, Raguzzini A, Villano DV, Cesqui E, Toti E, Catasta G, Serafini M. High fat meal increase of IL-17 is prevented by ingestion of fruit juice drink in healthy overweight subjects. *Curr Pharm Des.* 2012;18(1):85-90.

Perrelli A, Goitre L, Salzano AM, Moglia A, Scaloni A, Retta SF. Biological Activities, Health Benefits, and Therapeutic Properties of Avenanthramides: From Skin Protection to Prevention and Treatment of Cerebrovascular Diseases. *Oxid Med Cell Longev.* 2018:6015351.

Petsiou EI, Mitrou PI, Raptis SA, Dimitriadis GD. Effect and mechanisms of action of vinegar on glucose metabolism, lipid profile, and body weight. *Nutr Rev.* 2014;72(10):651-61.

Pittler MH, Ernst E. Dietary supplements for body-weight reduction: a systematic review. *Am J Clin Nutr.* 2004;79(4):529-36.

Pol K, de Graaf C, Meyer D, Mars M. The efficacy of daily snack replacement with oligofructose-enriched granola bars in overweight and obese adults: a 12-week randomised controlled trial. *Br J Nutr.* 2018;119(9):1076-1086.

Popp CJ, Beasley JM, Yi SS, Hu L, Wylie-Rosett J. A cross-sectional analysis of dietary protein intake and body composition among Chinese Americans. *J Nutr Sci.* 2019;8:e4.

Potu BK, Rao MS, Nampurath GK, Chamallamudi MR, Prasad K, Nayak SR, Dharmavarapu PK, Kedage V, Bhat KM. Evidence-based assessment of antiosteoporotic activity of petroleum-ether extract of *Cissus quadrangularis* Linn. On ovariectomy-induced osteoporosis. *Ups J Med Sci.* 2009;114(3):140-8.

Pourmasoumi M, Hadi A, Rafie N, Najafgholizadeh A, Mohammadi H, Rouhani MH. The effect of ginger supplementation on lipid profile: A systematic review and meta-analysis of clinical trials. *Phytomedicine.* 2018;43:28-36.

Preuss HG, Rao CV, Garis R, Bramble JD, Ohia SE, Bagchi M, Bagchi D. An overview of the safety and efficacy of a novel, natural(-)-hydroxycitric acid extract (HCA-SX) for weight management. *J Med.* 2004;35(1-6):33-48.

Quatela A, Callister R, Patterson AJ, McEvoy M, MacDonald-Wicks LK. Breakfast Cereal Consumption and Obesity Risk amongst the Mid-Age Cohort of the Australian Longitudinal Study on Women's Health. *Healthcare* (Basel). 2017;5(3). pii: E49.

Raghow R. Circadian rhythms of hormone secretion and obesity. *World J Diabetes*. 2018;9(11):195-198. doi: 10.4239/wjd.v9.i11.195.

Ranasinghe P, Jayawardana R, Galappaththy P, Constantine GR, de Vas Gunawardana N, Katulanda P. Efficacy and safety of 'true' cinnamon (*Cinnamomum zeylanicum*) as a pharmaceutical agent in diabetes: a systematic review and meta-analysis. *Diabet Med*. 2012;29(12):1480-92.

Rao PV, Gan SH. Cinnamon: a multifaceted medicinal plant. *Evid Based Complement Alternat Med*. 2014;2014:642942.

Rasane P, Jha A, Sabikhi L, Kumar A, Unnikrishnan VS. Nutritional advantages of oats and opportunities for its processing as value added foods - a review. *J Food Sci Technol*. 2015;52(2):662-75.

Reimer RA, Willis HJ, Tunnicliffe JM, Park H, Madsen KL, Soto-Vaca A. Inulin-type fructans and whey protein both modulate appetite but only fructans alter gut microbiota in adults with overweight/obesity: A randomized controlled trial. *Mol Nutr Food Res*. 2017;61(11):10.1002/ mnfr.201700484. doi:10.1002/mnfr.201700484.

Reinbach HC, Smeets A, Martinussen T, Møller P, Westerterp-Plantenga MS. Effects of capsaicin, green tea and CH-19 sweet pepper on appetite and energy intake in humans in negative and positive energy balance. *Clin Nutr*. 2009;28(3):260-5.

Reinbach HC, Smeets A, Martinussen T, Møller P, Westerterp-Plantenga MS. Effects of capsaicin, green tea and CH-19 sweet pepper on appetite and energy intake in humans in negative and positive energy balance. *Clin Nutr*. 2009;28(3):260-5.

Ren GY, Chen CY, Chen GC, Chen WG, Pan A, Pan CW, Zhang YH, Qin LQ, Chen LH. Effect of Flaxseed Intervention on Inflammatory Marker C-Reactive Protein: A Systematic Review and Meta-Analysis of Randomized Controlled Trials. *Nutrients*. 2016;8(3):136.

Ren GY, Chen CY, Chen GC, Chen WG, Pan A, Pan CW, Zhang YH, Qin LQ, Chen LH. Effect of Flaxseed Intervention on Inflammatory Marker C-Reactive Protein: A Systematic Review and Meta-Analysis of Randomized Controlled Trials. *Nutrients.* 2016;8(3):136.

Rendina E, Hembree KD, Davis MR, Marlow D, Clarke SL, Halloran BP, Lucas EA, Smith BJ. Dried plum's unique capacity to reverse bone loss and alter bone metabolism in postmenopausal osteoporosis model. *PLoS One.* 2013;8(3):e60569.

Rendón-Huerta JA, Juárez-Flores B, Pinos-Rodríguez JM, Aguirre-Rivera JR, Delgado-Portales RE. Effects of different sources of fructans on body weight, blood metabolites and fecal bacteria in normal and obese non-diabetic and diabetic rats. *Plant Foods Hum Nutr.* 2012;67(1):64-70.

Rhee Y, Brunt A. Flaxseed supplementation improved insulin resistance in obese glucose intolerant people: a randomized crossover design. *Nutr J.* 2011;10:44. doi: 10.1186/1475-2891-10-44.

Ribeiro C, Dourado G, Cesar T. Orange juice allied to a reduced-calorie diet results in weight loss and ameliorates obesity-related biomarkers: A randomized controlled trial. *Nutrition.* 2017;38:13-19.

Ribeiro DC, Pereira AD, da Silva PC, dos Santos Ade S, de Santana FC, Boueri BF, Pessanha CR, de Abreu MD, Mancini-Filho J, da Silva EM, do Nascimento-Saba CC, da Costa CA, Boaventura GT. Flaxseed flour (*Linum usitatissimum*) consumption improves bone quality and decreases the adipocyte area of lactating rats in the post-weaning period. *Int J Food Sci Nutr.* 2016;67(1):29-34.

Ricci E, Viganò P, Cipriani S, Somigliana E, Chiaffarino F, Bulfoni A, Parazzini F. Coffee and caffeine intake and male infertility: a systematic review. *Nutr J.* 2017;16(1):37.

Rico D, Martín-Diana AB, Martínez-Villaluenga C, Aguirre L, Silván JM, Dueñas M, De Luis DA, Lasa A. *In vitro* approach for evaluation of carob by-products as source bioactive ingredients with potential to attenuate metabolic syndrome (MetS). Heliyon. 2019;5(1):e01175. doi: 10.1016/j.heliyon.2019.e01175.

Ríos-Hoyo A, Gutiérrez-Salmeán G. New Dietary Supplements for Obesity: What We Currently Know. *Curr Obes Rep.* 2016;5(2):262-70.

Roberfroid MB. Concepts in functional foods: the case of inulin and oligofructose. *J Nutr.* 1999;129(7 Suppl):1398S-401S.

Roberts AT, Martin CK, Liu Z, Amen RJ, Woltering EA, Rood JC, Caruso MK, Yu Y, Xie H, Greenway FL. The safety and efficacy of a dietary herbal supplement and gallic acid for weight loss. *J Med Food.* 2007;10(1):184-8.

Robertson C, Archibald D, Avenell A, Douglas F, Hoddinott P, van Teijlingen E,Boyers D, Stewart F, Boachie C, Fioratou E, Wilkins D, Street T, Carroll P, Fowler C. Systematic reviews of and integrated report on the quantitative, qualitative and economic evidence base for the management of obesity in men. *Health Technol Assess.* 2014;18(35):v-vi, xxiii-xxix, 1-424.

Rodrigues EL, Marcelino G, Silva GT, Figueiredo PS, Garcez WS, Corsino J, Guimarães RCA, Freitas KC. Nutraceutical and medicinal potential of the *Morus* species in metabolic dysfunctions. *Int J Mol Sci.* 2019;20(2). pii: E301.

Rogovik AL, Goldman RD. Should weight-loss supplements be used for pediatric obesity? *Can Fam Physician.* 2009;55(3):257-9.

Rojas E, Bermúdez V, Motlaghzadeh Y, Mathew J, Fidilio E, Faria J, Rojas J, de Bravo MC, Contreras J, Mantilla LP, Angarita L, Sepúlveda PA, Kuzmar I. *Stevia rebaudiana* bertoni and its effects in human disease: emphasizing its role in inflammation, atherosclerosis and metabolic syndrome. *Curr Nutr Rep.* 2018.doi: 10.1007/s13668-018-0228-z.

Rollyson WD, Stover CA, Brown KC, Perry HE, Stevenson CD, McNees CA, Ball JG, Valentovic MA, Dasgupta P. Bioavailability of capsaicin and its implications for drug delivery. *J Control Release.* 2014;196:96-105.

Roongpisuthipong C, Kantawan R, Roongpisuthipong W. Reduction of adipose tissue and body weight: effect of water-soluble calcium hydroxycitrate in *Garcinia atroviridis* on the short-term treatment of obese women in Thailand. *Asia Pac J Clin Nutr.* 2007;16(1):25-9.

Ross SM. African mango (IGOB131): a proprietary seed extract of *Irvingia gabonensis* is found to be effective in reducing body weight and improving metabolic parameters in overweight humans. *Holist Nurs Pract.* 2011;25(4):215-7.

Rothenberg DO, Zhou C, Zhang L. A Review on the Weight-Loss Effects of Oxidized Tea Polyphenols. *Molecules.* 2018;23(5). pii: E1176.

Rtibi K, Selmi S, Grami D, Amri M, Eto B, El-Benna J, Sebai H, Marzouki L. Chemical constituents and pharmacological actions of carob pods and leaves (*Ceratonia siliqua* L.) on the gastrointestinal tract: A review. *Biomed Pharmacother.* 2017;93:522-528. doi: 10.1016/j.biopha.2017.06.088.

Ruiz-Roso B, Quintela JC, de la Fuente E, Haya J, Pérez-Olleros L. Insoluble carob fiber rich in polyphenols lowers total and LDL cholesterol in hypercholesterolemic sujects. *Plant Foods Hum Nutr.* 2010;65(1):50-6. doi: 10.1007/s11130-009-0153-9.

Ruiz-Ruiz JC, Moguel-Ordoñez YB, Segura-Campos MR. Biological activity of *Stevia rebaudiana* Bertoni and their relationship to health. *Crit Rev Food Sci Nutr.* 2017;57(12):2680-90.

Russell WR, Baka A, Björck I, Delzenne N, Gao D, Griffiths HR, Hadjilucas E, Juvonen K, Lahtinen S, Lansink M, Loon LV, Mykkänen H, Östman E, Riccardi G, Vinoy S, Weickert MO. Impact of Diet Composition on Blood Glucose Regulation. *Crit Rev Food Sci Nutr.* 2016;56(4):541-90.

Saito M, Ueno M, Ogino S, Kubo K, Nagata J, Takeuchi M. High dose of *Garcinia cambogia* is effective in suppressing fat accumulation in developing male Zucker obese rats, but highly toxic to the testis. *Food Chem Toxicol.* 2005;43(3):411-9.

Sakakibara S, Yamauchi T, Oshima Y, Tsukamoto Y, Kadowaki T. Acetic acid activates hepatic AMPK and reduces hyperglycemia in diabetic KK-A(y) mice. *Biochem Biophys Res Commun.* 2006;344(2):597-604.

Saldanha LG, Dwyer JT, Betz JM. Culinary Spice Plants in Dietary Supplement Products and Tested in Clinical Trials. *Adv Nutr.* 2016;7(2):343-8.

Samuel P, Ayoob KT, Magnuson BA, Wölwer-Rieck U, Jeppesen PB, Rogers PJ, Rowland I, Mathews R. Stevia Leaf to Stevia Sweetener:

Exploring Its Science, Benefits, and Future Potential. *J Nutr.* 2018;148(7):1186S-1205S.

Sanati S, Razavi BM, Hosseinzadeh H. A review of the effects of Capsicum annuum L. and its constituent, capsaicin, in metabolic syndrome. *Iran J Basic Med Sci.* 2018;21(5):439-48.

Sanchez M, Darimont C, Panahi S, Drapeau V, Marette A, Taylor VH, Doré J, Tremblay A. Effects of a Diet-Based Weight-Reducing Program with Probiotic Supplementation on Satiety Efficiency, Eating Behaviour Traits, and Psychosocial Behaviours in Obese Individuals. *Nutrients.* 2017;9(3). pii: E284.

Santos HO, da Silva GAR. To what extent does cinnamon administration improve the glycemic and lipid profiles? *Clin Nutr ESPEN.* 2018;27:1-9.

Saravanan G, Ponmurugan P, Deepa MA, Senthilkumar B. Anti-obesity action of gingerol: effect on lipid profile, insulin, leptin, amylase and lipase in male obese rats induced by a high-fat diet. *J Sci Food Agric.* 2014;94(14):2972-7.

Sarriá B, Martínez-López S, Sierra-Cinos JL, García-Diz L, Mateos R, Bravo-Clemente L. Regularly consuming a green/roasted coffee blend reduces the risk of metabolic syndrome. *Eur J Nutr.* 2018;57(1):269-278.

Sawangjit R, Puttarak P, Saokaew S, Chaiyakunapruk N. Efficacy and Safety of *Cissus quadrangularis* L. in Clinical Use: A Systematic Review and Meta-analysis of Randomized Controlled Trials. *Phytother Res.* 2017;31(4):555-67.

Sayin MR, Karabag T, Dogan SM, Akpinar I, Aydin M. A case of acute myocardial infarction due to the use of cayenne pepper pills. *Wien Klin Wochenschr.* 2012;124(7-8):285-7.

Schutz Y. Protein turnover, ureagenesis and gluconeogenesis. *Int J Vitam Nutr Res.* 2011;81(2-3):101-7.

Schwarz JM, Clearfield M, Mulligan K. Conversion of Sugar to Fat: Is Hepatic de Novo Lipogenesis Leading to Metabolic Syndrome and Associated Chronic Diseases? *J Am Osteopath Assoc.* 2017;117(8):520-527.

Scott AD, Orsi A, Ward C, Bradford R. Genotoxicity testing of a Hoodia gordonii extract. *Food Chem Toxicol.* 2012;50 (Suppl 1):S34-40.

Seitz J, Belheouane M, Schulz N, Dempfle A, Baines JF, Herpertz-Dahlmann B. The impact of starvation on the microbiome and gut-brain interaction in anorexia nervosa. *Front Endocrinol* (Lausanne). 2019;10:41.

Semwal RB, Semwal DK, Combrinck S, Viljoen AM. Gingerols and shogaols: Important nutraceutical principles from ginger. *Phytochemistry.* 2015;117:554-68.

Semwal RB, Semwal DK, Vermaak I, Viljoen A. A comprehensive scientific overview of Garcinia cambogia. *Fitoterapia.* 2015;102:134-48.

Seyithanoğlu M, Öner-İyidoğan Y, Doğru-Abbasoğlu S, Tanrıkulu-Küçük S, Koçak H, Beyhan-Özdaş Ş, Koçak-Toker N. The effect of dietary curcumin and capsaicin on hepatic fetuin-A expression and fat accumulation in rats fed on a high-fat diet. *Arch Physiol Biochem.* 2016;122(2):94-102.

Shang HM, Zhou HZ, Yang JY, Li R, Song H, Wu HX. In vitro and in vivo antioxidant activities of inulin. *PLoS One.* 2018;13(2):e0192273.

Shara M, Ohia SE, Yasmin T, Zardetto-Smith A, Kincaid A, Bagchi M, Chatterjee A, Bagchi D, Stohs SJ. Dose- and time-dependent effects of a novel (-)-hydroxycitric acid extract on body weight, hepatic and testicular lipid peroxidation, DNA fragmentation and histopathological data over a period of 90 days. *Mol Cell Biochem.* 2003;254(1-2):339-46.

Sharifi-Rad M, Varoni EM, Salehi B, Sharifi-Rad J, Matthews KR, Ayatollahi SA, Kobarfard F, Ibrahim SA, Mnayer D, Zakaria ZA, Sharifi-Rad M, Yousaf Z, Iriti M, Basile A, Rigano D. Plants of the Genus Zingiber as a Source of Bioactive Phytochemicals: From Tradition to Pharmacy. *Molecules.* 2017 Dec 4;22(12). pii: E2145.

Shishehbor F, Mansoori A, Shirani F. Vinegar consumption can attenuate postprandial glucose and insulin responses; a systematic review and meta-analysis of clinical trials. *Diabetes Res Clin Pract.* 2017;127:1-9.

Shivashankara AR, Azmidah A, Haniadka R, Rai MP, Arora R, Baliga MS. Dietary agents in the prevention of alcohol-induced hepatotoxicty: preclinical observations. *Food Funct.* 2012;3(2):101-9.

Shoaib M, Shehzad A, Omar M, Rakha A, Raza H, Sharif HR, Shakeel A, Ansari A, Niazi S. Inulin: Properties, health benefits and food applications. *Carbohydr Polym.* 2016;147:444-454.

Siddiqui FJ, Assam PN, de Souza NN, Sultana R, Dalan R, Chan ES. Diabetes Control: Is Vinegar a Promising Candidate to Help Achieve Targets? *J Evid Based Integr Med.* 2018;23:2156587217753004.

Silvester AJ, Aseer KR, Yun JW. Dietary polyphenols and their roles in fat browning. *J Nutr Biochem.* 2019;64:1-12.

Singh AK, Bishayee A, Pandey AK. Targeting Histone Deacetylases with Natural and Synthetic Agents: An Emerging Anticancer Strategy. *Nutrients.* 2018;10(6). pii: E731.

Singh KK, Mridula D, Rehal J, Barnwal P. Flaxseed: a potential source of food, feed and fiber. *Crit Rev Food Sci Nutr.* 2011;51(3):210-22.

Singh S, Singh G, Arya SK. Mannans: An overview of properties and application in food products. *Int J Biol Macromol.* 2018;119:79-95.

Skrypnik K, Suliburska J, Skrypnik D, Pilarski Ł, Reguła J, Bogdański P. The genetic basis of obesity complications. *Acta Sci Pol Technol Aliment.* 2017;16(1):83-91.

Smith C, Krygsman A. Hoodia gordonii extract targets both adipose and muscle tissue to achieve weight loss in rats. *J Ethnopharmacol.* 2014a;155(2):1284-90.

Smith C, Krygsman A. *Hoodia gordonii*: to eat, or not to eat. *J Ethnopharmacol.* 2014b;155(2):987-91.

Smith CE, Mollard RC, Luhovyy BL, Anderson GH. The effect of yellow pea protein and fibre on short-term food intake, subjective appetite and glycaemic response in healthy young men. *Br J Nutr.* 2012;108 Suppl 1:S74-S80.

Sood N, Baker WL, Coleman CI. Effect of glucomannan on plasma lipid and glucose concentrations, body weight, and blood pressure: systematic review and meta-analysis. *Am J Clin Nutr.* 2008;88(4):1167-75.

Souza SJ, Petrilli AA, Teixeira AM, Pontilho PM, Carioca AA, Luzia LA, Souza JM, Damasceno NR, Segurado AA, Rondó PH. Effect of chocolate and mate tea on the lipid profile of individuals with HIV/AIDS on antiretroviral therapy: A clinical trial. *Nutrition.* 2017;43-44:61-8.

Srinivasan K. Antioxidant potential of spices and their active constituents. *Crit Rev Food Sci Nutr.* 2014;54(3):352-72.

Srinivasan K. Biological Activities of Red Pepper (*Capsicum annuum*) and Its Pungent Principle Capsaicin: A Review. *Crit Rev Food Sci Nutr.* 2016;56(9):1488-500.

Stacewicz-Sapuntzakis M. Dried plums and their products: composition and health effects--an updated review. *Crit Rev Food Sci Nutr.* 2013;53(12):1277-302.

Stanko P. Možnosti uplatnenia výživových doplnkov u pacientov s nadváhou a obezitou [Possible application of food additives in patients with overweight and obesity]. *Via practica* 2008;5:131-134.

Steinglass JE, Walsh BT. Neurobiological model of the persistence of anorexia nervosa. *J Eat Disord.* 2016;4:19.

Stohs SJ, Badmaev V. A Review of Natural Stimulant and Non-stimulant Thermogenic Agents. *Phytother Res.* 2016;30(5):732-40.

Stohs SJ, Ray SD. A review and evaluation of the efficacy and safety of *Cissus quadrangularis* extracts. *Phytother Res.* 2013;27(8):1107-14.

Stoner GD. Ginger: is it ready for prime time? *Cancer Prev Res* (Phila). 2013 Apr;6(4):257-62.

Støving RK. Mechanisms in Endocrinology: Anorexia nervosa and endocrinology: a clinical update. *Eur J Endocrinol.* 2019;180(1):R9-R27.

Suetonius GT. *Životopisy rímskych cisárov.* [*The life of the roman caesars*] Vydavateľstvo Spolku slovenských spisovateľov, Bratislava, 2010, 311 pp, ISBN 9788080614270.

Suiryanrayna MV, Ramana JV. A review of the effects of dietary organic acids fed to swine. *J Anim Sci Biotechnol.* 2015;6:45.

Sun BY, Zhang B, Lin ZJ, Li LY, Wang HP, Zhou J. [Chicory extract's influence on gut bacteria of abdominal obesity rat]. *Zhongguo Zhong Yao Za Zhi.* 2014;39(11):2081-5.

Sun J, Chen P. Ultra high-performance liquid chromatography with high-resolution mass spectrometry analysis of African mango (*Irvingia gabonensis*) seeds, extract, and related dietary supplements. *J Agric Food Chem.* 2012;60(35):8703-9.

Sun X, Yamasaki M, Katsube T, Shiwaku K. Effects of quercetin derivatives from mulberry leaves: Improved gene expression related hepatic lipid and glucose metabolism in short-term high-fat fed mice. *Nutr Res Pract.* 2015;9(2):137-43.

Sung J, Ho CT, Wang Y. Preventive mechanism of bioactive dietary foods on obesity-related inflammation and diseases. *Food Funct.* 2018; 9(12):6081-95.

Tabrizi R, Saneei P, Lankarani KB, Akbari M, Kolahdooz F, Esmaillzadeh A, Nadi-Ravandi S, Mazoochi M, Asemi Z. The effects of caffeine intake on weight loss: a systematic review and dose-response meta-analysis of randomized controlled trials. *Crit Rev Food Sci Nutr.* 2019;59(16):2688-2696.

Taghizadeh M, Farzin N, Taheri S, Mahlouji M, Akbari H, Karamali F, Asemi Z. The Effect of Dietary Supplements Containing Green Tea, Capsaicin and Ginger Extracts on Weight Loss and Metabolic Profiles in Overweight Women: A Randomized Double-Blind Placebo-Controlled Clinical Trial. *Ann Nutr Metab.* 2017;70(4):277-85.

Tajik N, Tajik M, Mack I, Enck P. The potential effects of chlorogenic acid, the main phenolic components in coffee, on health: a comprehensive review of the literature. *Eur J Nutr.* 2017;56(7):2215-2244.

Tavares Toscano L, Tavares Toscano L, Leite Tavares R, da Oliveira Silva CS, Silva AS. Chia induces clinically discrete weight loss and improves lipid profile only in altered previous values. *Nutr Hosp.* 2014;31(3):1176-82.

Tchoundjeu Z, Atangana, AR. Irvingia gabonensis (Aubry-Lecomte ex O'Rorke) Baill. In: *Plant Resources of Tropical Africa* (PROTA) (Eds. van der Vossen HAM, Mkamilo GS); 2007, Wageningen, Netherlands.

Tenk J, Mátrai P, Hegyi P, Rostás I, Garami A, Szabó I, Hartmann P, Pétervári E, Czopf L, Hussain A, Simon M, Szujó S, Balaskó M. Perceived stress correlates with visceral obesity and lipid parameters of the metabolic syndrome: A systematic review and meta-analysis. *Psychoneuroendocrinology.* 2018;95:63-73.

Tremblay A, Arguin H, Panahi S. Capsaicinoids: a spicy solution to the management of obesity? *Int J Obes* (Lond). 2016;40(8):1198-204.

Tsoukalas M, Muller CD, Lobstein A, Urbain A. Pregnane Glycosides from *Cynanchum marnierianum* Stimulate GLP-1 Secretion in STC-1 Cells. *Planta Med.* 2016;82(11-12):992-9.

Tunnicliffe JM, Shearer J. Coffee, glucose homeostasis, and insulin resistance: physiological mechanisms and mediators. *Appl Physiol Nutr Metab.* 2008;33(6):1290-300.

Türközü D, Tek NA. A minireview of effects of green tea on energy expenditure. *Crit Rev Food Sci Nutr.* 2017;57(2):254-8.

Ulbricht C, Chao W, Nummy K, Rusie E, Tanguay-Colucci S, Iannuzzi CM, Plammoottil JB, Varghese M, Weissner W. Chia (*Salvia hispanica*): a systematic review by the natural standard research collaboration. *Rev Recent Clin Trials.* 2009;4(3):168-74.

Unachukwu UJ, Ahmed S, Kavalier A, Lyles JT, Kennelly EJ. White and green teas (*Camellia sinensis* var. sinensis): variation in phenolic, methylxanthine, and antioxidant profiles. *J Food Sci.* 2010;75(6):C541-8.

Unno K, Furushima D, Hamamoto S, Iguchi K, Yamada H, Morita A, Horie H, Nakamura Y. Stress-Reducing Function of Matcha Green Tea in Animal Experiments and Clinical Trials. *Nutrients.* 2018;10(10). pii: E1468.

Uragoda CG. Asthma and other symptoms in cinnamon workers. *Br J Ind Med.* 1984;41(2):224-7.

Urban JD, Carakostas MC, Taylor SL. Steviol glycoside safety: are highly purified steviol glycoside sweeteners food allergens? *Food Chem Toxicol.* 2015;75:71-8.

Utsunomiya H, Yamakawa T, Kamei J, Kadonosono K, Tanaka S. Antihyperglycemic effects of plum in a rat model of obesity and type 2 diabetes, Wistar fatty rat. *Biomed Res.* 2005;26(5):193-200.

Valdivia-López MÁ, Tecante A. Chia (*Salvia hispanica*): A Review of Native Mexican Seed and its Nutritional and Functional Properties. *Adv Food Nutr Res.* 2015;75:53-75.

van Heerden FR, Marthinus Horak R, Maharaj VJ, Vleggaar R, Senabe JV, Gunning PJ. An appetite suppressant from Hoodia species. *Phytochemistry.* 2007;68(20):2545-53.

Van Hul M, Geurts L, Plovier H, Druart C, Everard A, Ståhlman M, Rhimi M, Chira K, Teissedre PL, Delzenne NM, Maguin E, Guilbot A, Brochot A, Gérard P, Bäckhed F, Cani PD. Reduced obesity, diabetes, and steatosis upon cinnamon and grape pomace are associated with changes in gut microbiota and markers of gut barrier. *Am J Physiol Endocrinol Metab.* 2018;314(4):E334-E352.

Varghese S, Kubatka P, Rodrigo L, Gazdikova K, Caprnda M, Fedotova J, Zulli A, Kruzliak P, Büsselberg D. Chili pepper as a body weight-loss food. *Int J Food Sci Nutr.* 2017;68(4):392-401.

Vázquez Cisneros LC, López-Uriarte P, López-Espinoza A, Navarro Meza M, Espinoza-Gallardo AC, Guzmán Aburto MB. Effects of green tea and its epigallocatechin (EGCG) content on body weight and fat mass in humans: a systematic review. *Nutr Hosp.* 2017;34(3):731-7.

Vermaak I, Hamman JH, Viljoen AM. Hoodia gordonii: an up-to-date review of a commercially important anti-obesity plant. *Planta Med.* 2011;77(11):1149-60.

Vettori A, Pompucci G, Paolini B, Del Ciondolo I, Bressan S, Dundar M, Kenanoğlu S, Unfer V, Bertelli M; Geneob Project. Genetic background, nutrition and obesity: a review. *Eur Rev Med Pharmacol Sci.* 2019;23(4):1751-1761.

Vieira-Brock PL, Vaughan BM, Vollmer DL. Thermogenic Blend Alone or in Combination with Whey Protein Supplement Stimulates Fat Metabolism and Improves Body Composition in Mice. *Pharmacognosy Res.* 2018;10(1):37-43.

Vollmannová A., Musilová J, Urminská D et al. *Chémia potravín* [*Chemistry of food*]. Slovenská poľnohospodárska univerzita v Nitre, Nitra, 2018, 543 s.

Vuksan V, Jenkins AL, Brissette C, Choleva L, Jovanovski E, Gibbs AL, Bazinet RP, Au-Yeung F, Zurbau A, Ho HV, Duvnjak L, Sievenpiper JL, Josse RG, Hanna A. Salba-chia (*Salvia hispanica* L.) in the treatment of overweight and obese patients with type 2 diabetes: A double-blind randomized controlled trial. *Nutr Metab Cardiovasc Dis.* 2017;27(2):138-146.

Wallace TC. Dried Plums, Prunes and Bone Health: A Comprehensive Review. *Nutrients.* 2017;9(4). pii: E401.

Wanders AJ, van den Borne JJ, de Graaf C, Hulshof T, Jonathan MC, Kristensen M, Mars M, Schols HA, Feskens EJ. Effects of dietary fibre on subjective appetite, energy intake and body weight: a systematic review of randomized controlled trials. *Obes Rev.* 2011;12(9):724-39.

Wang J, Ke W, Bao R, Hu X, Chen F. Beneficial effects of ginger *Zingiber officinale* Roscoe on obesity and metabolic syndrome: a review. *Ann N Y Acad Sci.* 2017 Jun;1398(1):83-98.

Weiss DJ, Anderton CR. Determination of catechins in matcha green tea by micellar electrokinetic chromatography. *J Chromatogr A.* 2003;1011(1-2):173-80.

Whelan AM, Jurgens TM, Szeto V. Case report. Efficacy of Hoodia for weight loss: is there evidence to support the efficacy claims? *J Clin Pharm Ther.* 2010;35(5):609-12.

Whitfield P, Parry-Strong A, Walsh E, Weatherall M, Krebs JD. The effect of a cinnamon-, chromium- and magnesium-formulated honey on glycaemic control, weight loss and lipid parameters in type 2 diabetes: an open-label cross-over randomised controlled trial. *Eur J Nutr.* 2016;55(3):1123-31.

Whiting S, Derbyshire EJ, Tiwari B. Could capsaicinoids help to support weight management? A systematic review and meta-analysis of energy intake data. *Appetite.* 2014;73:183-8.

Willems MET, Şahin MA, Cook MD. Matcha green tea drinks enhance fat oxidation during brisk walking in females. *Int J Sport Nutr Exerc Metab.* 2018;28(5):536-41.

Williams PG. The benefits of breakfast cereal consumption: a systematic review of the evidence base. *Adv Nutr.* 2014;5(5):636S-673S.

Williamson EM. *Potter's Herbal Cyclopaedia.* The autoritative reference work on plants with a known medicinal use. Saffron Walden, The C. W. Daniel Company Limited 2003; 67.

Williamson G, Dionisi F, Renouf M. Flavanols from green tea and phenolic acids from coffee: critical quantitative evaluation of the pharmacokinetic data in humans after consumption of single doses of beverages. *Mol Nutr Food Res.* 2011;55(6):864-73.

Wilson B, Whelan K. Prebiotic inulin-type fructans and galacto-oligosaccharides: definition, specificity, function, and application in gastrointestinal disorders. *J Gastroenterol Hepatol.* 2017;32 Suppl 1:64-68.

Wolf A, Bray GA, Popkin BM. A short history of beverages and how our body treats them. *Obes Rev.* 2008;9(2):151-64.

Wong LP, Klemmer PJ. Severe lactic acidosis associated with juice of the mangosteen fruit *Garcinia mangostana. Am J Kidney Dis.* 2008;51(5):829-33.

Wu T, Tang Q, Gao Z, Yu Z, Song H, Zheng X, Chen W. Blueberry and mulberry juice prevent obesity development in C57BL/6 mice. *PLoS One.* 2013;8(10):e77585.

Xie C, Cui L, Zhu J, Wang K, Sun N, Sun C. Coffee consumption and risk of hypertension: a systematic review and dose-response meta-analysis of cohort studies. *J Hum Hypertens.* 2018;32(2):83-93.

Xu H, Wang Y, Yuan Y, Zhang X, Zuo X, Cui L, Liu Y, Chen W, Su N, Wang H, Yan F, Li X, Wang T, Xiao S. Gender differences in the protective effects of green tea against amnestic mild cognitive impairment in the elderly Han population. *Neuropsychiatr Dis Treat.* 2018;14:1795-1801.

Yamada T, Hida H, Yamada Y. Chemistry, physiological properties, and microbial production of hydroxycitric acid. *Appl Microbiol Biotechnol.* 2007;75(5):977-82.

Yamashita H. Biological Function of Acetic Acid-Improvement in Obesity and Glucose Tolerance by Acetic Acid in Type 2 Diabetic Rats. Crit *Rev Food Sci Nutr.* 2016;56 Suppl 1:S171-5.

Yang CS, Wang H, Sheridan ZP. Studies on prevention of obesity, metabolic syndrome, diabetes, cardiovascular diseases and cancer by tea. *J Food Drug Anal.* 2018;26(1):1-13.

Yang CS, Zhang J, Zhang L, Huang J, Wang Y. Mechanisms of body weight reduction and metabolic syndrome alleviation by tea. *Mol Nutr Food Res.* 2016;60(1):160-74.

Yang HJ, Kim MJ, Kang ES, Kim DS, Park S. Red mulberry fruit aqueous extract and silk proteins accelerate acute ethanol metabolism and promote the anti-oxidant enzyme systems in rats. *Mol Med Rep.* 2018;18(1):1197-1205.

Yashin A, Yashin Y, Wang JY, Nemzer B. Antioxidant and Antiradical Activity of Coffee. *Antioxidants* (Basel). 2013;2(4):230-45.

Yasueda A, Ito T, Maeda K. Review: Evidence-based Clinical Research of Anti-obesity Supplements in Japan. *Immunol Endocr Metab Agents Med Chem.* 2013;13(3):185-195.

Yimam M, Jiao P, Hong M, Brownell L, Lee YC, Hyun EJ, Kim HJ, Kim TW, Nam JB, Kim MR, Jia Q. Appetite suppression and antiobesity effect of a botanical composition composed of *Morus alba*, Yerba mate, and Magnolia officinalis. *J Obes.* 2016;2016:4670818.

Yodyingyuad V, Bunyawong S. Effect of stevioside on growth and reproduction. *Hum Reprod.* 1991;6(1):158-65.

Yoshida M, Ono H, Mori Y, Chuda Y, Mori M. Oxygenation of bisphenol A to quinones by polyphenol oxidase in vegetables. *J Agric Food* Chem. 2002;50(15):4377-81.

Yuan Q, Zhao L. The Mulberry (Morus alba L.) Fruit-A Review of Characteristic Components and Health Benefits. *J Agric Food Chem.* 2017;65(48):10383-94.

Zalewski BM, Chmielewska A, Szajewska H. The effect of glucomannan on body weight in overweight or obese children and adults: a systematic review of randomized controlled trials. *Nutrition.* 2015;31(3):437-42.

Zamora Navarro S, Pérez-Llamas F. Errors and myths in feeding and nutrition: impact on the problems of obesity. *Nutr Hosp.* 2013;28 Suppl 5:81-8.

Zanzer YC, Plaza M, Dougkas A, Turner C, Östman E. Black pepper-based beverage induced appetite-suppressing effects without altering postprandial glycaemia, gut and thyroid hormones or gastrointestinal well-being: a randomized crossover study in healthy subjects. *Food Funct.* 2018;9(5):2774-86.

Zeni ALB, Moreira TD, Dalmagro AP, Camargo A, Bini LA, Simionatto EL, Scharf DR. Evaluation of phenolic compounds and lipid-lowering effect of *Morus nigra* leaves extract. *An Acad Bras Cienc.* 2017;89(4):2805-2815.

Zero DT, Lussi A. Erosion--chemical and biological factors of importance to the dental practitioner. *Int Dent J.* 2005;55(4 Suppl 1):285-90.

Zhang H, Ma ZF, Luo X, Li X. Effects of Mulberry Fruit (*Morus alba* L.) Consumption on Health Outcomes: A Mini-Review. *Antioxidants (Basel).* 2018;7(5). pii: E69.

Zhang S, Ma X, Zhang L, Sun H, Liu X. Capsaicin Reduces Blood Glucose by Increasing Insulin Levels and Glycogen Content Better than Capsiate in Streptozotocin-Induced Diabetic Rats. *J Agric Food Chem.* 2017;65(11):2323-30.

Zhang S, Ma Y, Li J, Ma J, Yu B, Xie X. Molecular matchmaking between the popular weight-loss herb *Hoodia gordonii* and GPR119, a potential drug target for metabolic disorder. *Proc Natl Acad Sci USA.* 2014;111(40):14571-6.

Zhong L, Furne JK, Levitt MD. An extract of black, green, and mulberry teas causes malabsorption of carbohydrate but not of triacylglycerol in healthy volunteers. *Am J Clin Nutr.* 2006;84(3):551-5.

Zhou Y, Li Y, Zhou T, Zheng J, Li S, Li HB. Dietary Natural Products for Prevention and Treatment of Liver Cancer. *Nutrients.* 2016;8(3):156.

Zoué LT, Bédikou ME, Faulet BM, Gonnety JT, Niamké SL. Characterisation of a highly saturated Irvingia gabonensis seed kernel oil with unusual linolenic acid content. *Food Sci Technol Int.* 2013;19(1):79-87.

Zubrzycki A, Cierpka-Kmiec K, Kmiec Z, Wronska A. The role of low-calorie diets and intermittent fasting in the treatment of obesity and type-2 diabetes. *J Physiol Pharmacol.* 2018;69(5). doi: 10.26402/jpp.2018.5.02.

Zunft HJ, Lüder W, Harde A, Haber B, Graubaum HJ, Koebnick C, Grünwald J. Carob pulp preparation rich in insoluble fibre lowers total and LDL cholesterol in hypercholesterolemic patients. *Eur J Nutr.* 2003;42(5):235-42.

WEBSITE LINKS

http://dni.skwww.plusden.sk/zena/chudnutie/dieta-tento-tyzden/jablcny-ocot-naozaj-roztopi-tuk-potvrdili-aj-vedci.html.

http://rx.travelweblog.net/categories/Weight%20Loss/Hoodia.

http://tn.nova.cz/clanek/pozor-na-kokosovy-olej-zpusobuje-nemoci-srdce-a-cev.html.

http://www.cajovnik.sk/caj-a-jeho-druhy.html

http://www.chineseherbshealing.com/mulberry-leaf/

http://www.krv.fapz.uniag.sk/plodiny/Ovos%20siaty.pdf

http://www.liecive.herba.sk/index.php/koncentraty/herbar/1443-lan-siaty

http://www.ncbi.nlm.nih.gov/books/NBK501824/

http://www.pluska.sk/izdravie/archiv/zdravie/prevratne-zistenia-kave-kolko-salok-denne-je-zdravych.html).

http://www.toxicology.cz/modules.php?name=News&file=article&sid=446.

http://www.tvnoviny.sk/my-zeny/1833478_zdravy-ako-bukovsky-kokosovy-olej-vseliek-alebo-lacny-klam.

http://www.vurv.sk/fileadmin/CVRV/subory/aktivity/2013/Ovos-Noc_vyskumnika_2012.pdf)

http://www.whfoods.com/genpage.php?tname=foodspice&dbid=35.
https://abc-dieta.sk/chudnutie-s-hroznom.html.
https://biopedia.sk/clovek/vyziva-a-metabolizmus .
https://botanic.sk/slovnik-pojmov/fermentace.
https://cs.wikipedia.org/wiki/Inulin.
https://en.wikipedia.org/wiki/Camellia_sinensis.
https://en.wikipedia.org/wiki/Capsicum.
https://en.wikipedia.org/wiki/Chia_seed.
https://en.wikipedia.org/wiki/Cissus_quadrangularis.
https://en.wikipedia.org/wiki/Hoodia_gordonii.
https://en.wikipedia.org/wiki/Konjac.
https://en.wikipedia.org/wiki/Lipid_metabolism.
https://en.wikipedia.org/wiki/List_of_Capsicum_cultivars
https://en.wikipedia.org/wiki/Plum.
https://en.wikipedia.org/wiki/Stevia.
https://en.wikipedia.org/wiki/Yac%C3%B3n.
https://en.wikipedia.org/wiki/Yerba_mate.
https://feminity.zoznam.sk/c/894853/zazvor-a-jeho-ucinky-zazrak-v-malom-mnozstve#ixzz5VdFVo4Yk
https://fitastyl.sk/clanky/vyziva/pravda-o-kokosovom-oleji-alebo-tuku-ak-chcete.
https://legionathletics.com/31-super-foods-super-charge-weight-loss/.
https://medaboutme.ru/obraz-zhizni/publikacii/stati/pohudenie/9_faktov_pro_zhir_na_nashem_tele/.
https://ndb.nal.usda.gov/ndb/search/list?qlookup=12006&format=Full.
https://referaty.aktuality.sk/popis-a-pestovanie-caju/referat-16844.
https://schudnut-ako.webnode.sk/news/ako-schudnut-ovocie-vhodne-a-nevhodne-na-chudnutie-/.
https://schudnutie.peknetelo.eu/citron-pomelo-grep-mandarinka-pomaranc-chudnutie.html.
https://sk.simpleaslife.com/20118-side-effects-of-caffeine-free-hydroxycut.html
https://sk.simpleaslife.com/20805-side-effects-of-apple-cider-vinegar-tablets.html.

https://sk.thefreespiritedwoman.com/1888-5-side-effects-of-apple-cider-vinegar-nobody-told-you-about.

https://sk.wikipedia.org/wiki/Ľan_siaty.

https://soda.o2.sk/miesta/priroda-slovenska/zabudnute-poklady-slovenskych-zahrad-moruse/)

https://spalovace-tukov.heureka.sk/atp-hca-garcinia-cambogia-100-tabliet/specifikace/#section.

https://vysetrenie.zoznam.sk/cl/1000649/1500889/Oblubeny-zazvor-nie-je-pre-vsetkych--Vyvarujte-sa-ho-skor--ako-vam-ublizi-

https://vysetrenie.zoznam.sk/cl/1000654/1372046/Skorica-a-jej-ucinky--Pozitivne--ale-i-negativne.

https://wanda.pluska.sk/chudnutie-s-ananasom-zarucene/wellness-a-fit/chudnutie/539561.html.

https://www.biopoint.sk/p/165/zazvorovy-prasok-500g?gclid=CjwKCAjwyOreBRAYEiwAR2mSkjNOg-MbfTFQ0zvQEJVDI3T3jJEYVH-_G359Rm4YgcajcWgDjyC-PxoCQRQQAvD_BwE

https://www.ebay.com/p/Chicory-Root-Inulin-Powder-FOS-Soluble-Organic-Fiber-Prebiotic-Healthy-8oz-Pouch/1492138643?ef_id=CjwKCAjwyOreBRAYEiwAR2mSkhSY1yOQL2aLcRU26dh65N7vvzEDqbIHUzqGt_TQDoKNvjF4vhk0NhoCRxAQAvD_BwE:G:s

https://www.healthline.com/nutrition/apple-cider-vinegar-weight-loss#section7.

https://www.healthline.com/nutrition/benefits-of-plums-prunes#section2

https://www.healthline.com/nutrition/fiber-can-help-you-lose-weight#inflammation

https://www.healthline.com/nutrition/glucomannan#weight-loss

https://www.hlavnespravy.sk/krutym-hladom-trpi-vo-svete-podla-statistiky-viac-ako-100-milionov-ludi/1726018.

https://www.mayoclinic.org/healthy-lifestyle/nutrition-and-healthy-eating/in-depth/caffeine/art-20045678.

https://www.mirapa.cz/hca-pravda-o-garcinia-cambogia-kyselina-hydroxicitronova/.

Bibliography

https://www.namaximum.sk/kategoria/sacharidy/inulin/?gclid=CjwKCAjw
yOreBRAYEiwAR2mSkrnUIsxBJ06AADoUG_jGXVb_esoPz7H7Gb
v7yDG72oQY1xaBCxyRhxoC6ZQQAvD_BwE

https://www.namaximum.sk/kategoria/zdrave-potraviny/garcinia-
cambogia/?gclid=CjwKCAjw39reBRBJEiwAO1m0ObgY4FbhxCwk7
BVwNVBP1fLLWk_jXIzC9fQph2YMe3hQetVFBCqu7xoC_6gQAv
D_BwE.

https://www.nazdravie.sk/cakanka-obycajna/.

https://www.ncbi.nlm.nih.gov/books/NBK459168/

https://www.newnordic.ca/products/zuccarin-diet?variant=4339114934299

https://www.pluska.sk/zena/chudnutie/dieta-tento-tyzden/jednoduchy-
zazrak-pite-vodu-citronom-4-dni-zbavite-az-2-kilogramov.html.

https://www.rd.com/health/diet-weight-loss/cinnamon-weight-loss/.

https://www.recenzie-plus.sk/bioxyn/.

https://www.revolvy.com/page/Cinnamomum.

https://www.rexter.cz/rubriky/zajimavosti/ucinky-piti-kavy-na-nase-
zdravi_165.html.

https://www.rxlist.com/consumer_garcinia/drugs-condition.htm.

https://www.sciencedirect.com/topics/medicine-and-dentistry/gingerol

https://www.slovenskypacient.sk/kava-a-zdravie-desat-prinosov-kavy/

https://www.verywellhealth.com/the-benefits-of-cissus-quadrangularis-
88623.

https://www.webmd.com/vitamins/ai/ingredientmono-1250/white-
mulberry

https://www.webmd.com/vitamins/ai/ingredientmono-205/glucomannan

https://www.webmd.com/vitamins-supplements/ingredientreview-205-
glucomannan.aspx?drugid=205&drugname=glucomannan.

https://www.webmd.com/vitamins-supplements/ingredientreview-205-
glucomannan.aspx?drugid=205&drugname=glucomannan

https://www.zdravie.sk/clanok/56489/ovos-avena-sativa-jedna-z-
najzdravsich-obilnin

https://www.zdravieastyl.sk/potraviny-a-vyziva/193-sila-jablcneho-octu.

https://www.zdravieastyl.sk/prirodna-medicina/23-cakanka-obycajna.

https://zaujimavosti.net/blog/je-zelena-kava-podvod-alebo-naozaj-funguje-jej-efekt-pri-spalovani-tukov).
https://zdravoteka.sk/byliny/cakanka-obycajna/
https://zena.pravda.sk/zdravy-zivot/clanok/389822-garcinia-kambodzska-slubuje-ubytok-hmotnosti-naozaj/.

ABOUT THE AUTHOR

Alexander Sirotkin, PhD, DrSc, works as a professor at the Faculty of Natural Sciences of the Constantine the Philosopher University in Nitra. His current activities are focused on reproductive biology, endocrinology, biotechnology and intracellular signalling. He was an investigator of several national and European projects focused towards the influence of nutrition and plant molecules on physiological functions of animals and humans.

Alexander Sirotkin, DrSc, was born on February 13th 1954 in Leningrad, USSR. He studied biology at the Faculty of Biology, Leningrad State University (1970-1976). He worked as a Senior Research Scientist at the Research Institute of Animal Breeding and Genetics Leningrad-Pushkin (1976-1988) and a Senior Research Scientist at the International Laboratory for Biotechnology within the Research Institute of Animal Production Nitra (1988-1992) and a Senior Research Scientist and a Head of Laboratory at the Research Institute of Animal Production Nitra (1992-2015). Afterwards he in 2014 accepted a professorial position at the Faculty of Natural Sciences of the Constantine the Philosopher University in Nitra. He took part in numerous study and teaching stays abroad.

Results of his research have been published in more than 680 publications including 3 monographs, 3 university textbooks and 11 chapters in monographs and textbooks. His works have been cited more than 2 700 times. As a teacher, he has supervised 22 doctoral and 34 graduate students.

He is a board member of 7 international journals. He has received more than 10 national and international awards. He coordinated 13 international and national projects.

Reviewers:

Prof. Dr. Radoslav Omelka, PhD.
Prof. Ing. Adriana Kolesárová, PhD.

INDEX

A

Acacia mearnsii (Australian acacia), 98
Acanthopanax senticosus (Siberian ginseng), 98
Acanthopanax sessiliflorus, 98
Actinidia arguta (hardy kiwi), 98
adipocytes, 13, 14, 25, 28, 73, 109, 120, 133
adipose tissue, 5, 6, 8, 9, 10, 11, 13, 20, 56, 68, 69, 72, 73, 85, 86, 103, 105, 107, 136, 138, 148, 150, 157
adverse side-effects, iv, ix, 3, 22, 23, 26, 28, 29, 33, 35, 40, 44, 47, 51, 54, 55, 57, 60, 61, 64, 65, 69, 73, 77, 78, 81, 85, 86, 87, 89, 90, 92, 95, 97, 119, 123
Aesculus turbinata (Japanese horse-chestnut), 98
Agave angustifolia (Caribbean agave), 98
Agave potatorum (butterfly agave), 98
Agave potatorum (Butterfly agave), 98
aloe (*Aloe vera*), 97, 119
Alpinia officinarum (lesser galangal), 98
anorexia nervosa, 2, 12, 160, 162
antibodies, 11

antioxidant, 21, 22, 24, 25, 27, 29, 31, 39, 42, 45, 49, 51, 56, 67, 68, 76, 79, 84, 88, 91, 93, 94, 104, 108, 128, 131, 133, 134, 140, 149, 151, 152, 160, 162, 164, 168
apple, iv, v, ix, 3, 20, 21, 22, 23, 100, 107, 108, 110, 111, 114, 118, 119, 120, 123, 136, 139, 150, 171, 172
apple cider vinegar, iv, v, ix, 3, 20, 21, 22, 23, 107, 108, 118, 119, 123, 136, 139, 150
Araucaria angustifolia (Parana pine), 98
Arum palaestinum (black calla lily), 98
asparagus (*Asparagus officinalis*), 37, 97, 110, 120
Aster yomena (Kitam.) (field aster), 98
avocado, 114, 115, 118, 120

B

bacteria, 11, 31, 38, 39, 77, 82, 83, 91, 120, 156, 163
basal metabolism, 18
Benincasa hispida (winter melon, 99
Betula platyphylla (Japanese white birch or Siberian silver birch), 99

bitter, 37, 97, 119
black elder (*Sambucus nigra*), 97, 120
body mass index (BMI), 6, 9, 11, 40, 43
body weight, vi, 4, 5, 10, 17, 22, 23, 26, 28, 31, 32, 35, 36, 39, 43, 46, 50, 51, 52, 53, 55, 57, 58, 60, 61, 63, 64, 68, 69, 72, 74, 77, 78, 80, 85, 87, 92, 94, 97, 98, 107, 109, 110, 111, 113, 115, 127, 129, 131, 142, 143, 150, 153, 154, 156, 157, 158, 160, 161, 165, 166, 168, 169
bofutsushosan, 97, 115, 119, 120
bofutsushosan (*Pulvis ledebouriellae compositae*), 97, 115, 119, 120
Bofutsushosan Pulvis ledebouriellae compositae, 97, 115
Brassica nigra (black mustard), 99
breakfast, 10, 16, 62, 115, 125, 137, 139, 147, 155, 167
broccoli extract, 120
burning of fat, 8, 9, 18, 20, 22, 73, 89

C

calorie, 2, 10, 17, 20, 25, 35, 39, 55, 58, 59, 75, 80, 82, 86, 91, 92, 105, 108, 115, 117, 120, 127, 156, 170
Calotropis procera Aiton, 99
Camellia sinensis (tea plant), 82, 99, 129, 131, 133, 141, 142, 164
cancer, 1, 14, 25, 31, 34, 42, 49, 74, 76, 79, 84, 88, 162, 168, 169
Capparis decidua (karira), 99
Capsicum spp (hot and sweet peppers), vi, 48, 70, 99, 108, 118
Caralluma fimbriata Wall (cactus), 52, 99
carbohydrates, 4, 11, 14, 15, 21, 55, 61, 71, 75
cardiovascular and reproductive, 1
Carissa carandas (dogbane), 99
carob, iv, v, ix, 3, 23, 24, 25, 26, 118, 120, 123, 135, 142, 147, 156, 158, 170
carotenoids, 24, 70, 97, 120
carotenoids lutein and fucoxanthin, 120
Cassia siamea (Senna siamea, 99
Catha edulis (khat or qat), 99
Celastrus regelii =Trypterigium regelii (Regel's threewingnut), 99
chia, iv, v, ix, 3, 34, 35, 107, 108, 114, 118, 120, 123, 133, 147, 150, 153, 163, 164, 165, 166, 171
chicory, iv, v, ix, 3, 36, 37, 38, 39, 40, 118, 123, 144, 163, 172
chicory/inulin, 3, 118
chitosans, 97, 120
chitosans and pyruvates., 97, 120
cholesterols, 6
Chrysanthemum indicum (Indian chrysanthemum), 99
cinnamon, iv, v, ix, 3, 31, 32, 33, 107, 108, 118, 119, 123, 125, 134, 136, 138, 140, 142, 145, 146, 147, 148, 149, 150, 155, 159, 164, 165, 166, 173
circadian rhythms, 10, 16, 155
Cirsium setidens (gondre), 99
Cissus quadrangularis, iv, vi, ix, 87, 97, 109, 110, 123, 127, 131, 147, 149, 151, 154, 159, 162
Citrus depressa Hayata (shiikuwasha), 99
citrus flavonoids naringin and hesperidin, 120
Citrus unshiu (Satsuma Mandarin), 99
Clusia nemorosa (clusia), 99
coconut, 113, 119, 127, 135
coconut oil, 113, 119, 127, 135
Coffea arabica (Arabic coffee), v, 26, 99
coffee, iv, v, ix, 3, 26, 27, 28, 29, 30, 36, 62, 64, 93, 99, 104, 107, 108, 110, 118, 119, 123, 129, 130, 133, 134, 135, 140, 145, 151, 153, 156, 159, 163, 164, 167, 168
Coleous forskohlii, 97, 120
Coleous forskohlii and its molecule forskolin, 120

Index

common bean (*Phaseolus vulgaris*), 97, 100, 110, 119
Cosmos caudatus Kunth (Ulam raja), 99
Crataegus azarolus (Mediterranean medlar or azarole), 99
Crocus sativus (saffron), 99, 110, 167
Cudrania tricuspidata (Mandarin melon berry), 99
Curcuma longa (turmeric), 99

D

dandelion (*Taraxacum officinale*), 114, 115, 118, 120
diabetes, 1, 13, 21, 23, 27, 29, 32, 34, 39, 42, 45, 47, 49, 56, 59, 60, 62, 67, 71, 76, 78, 79, 81, 85, 89, 91, 92, 94, 108, 130, 144, 149, 155, 160, 161, 165, 166, 168, 170
diet, iv, 2, 4, 10, 11, 14, 17, 25, 32, 35, 66, 77, 105, 120, 127, 129, 130, 131, 132, 139, 140, 141, 146, 148, 150, 152, 156, 158, 159, 160, 173
digestibility, 11, 43, 128, 143
Dioscorea oppositifolia (Chinese yam), 99
Diospyros kaki (Japanese Persimmon – kaki), 99

E

Ecklonia cava, 99
Eclipta alba (false daisy), 99
Eisenia bicyclis (Arame – sea oak), 99
elder (*Sambucus nigra*), 97, 120
Eleusine indica (Indian goosegrass), 99
enzymes, 20, 25, 32, 37, 51, 58, 64, 67, 73, 77, 78, 82, 83, 91, 95, 107, 108, 152
Ephedra spp, 97
ephedrine, 97, 115, 119, 120
Eugenia caryophyllus (clove), 99
Euphorbia supina (Prostrate Spurge), 99

Evodiae Fructus = E. rutaecarpa (Evodia), 99

F

fasting, 14, 16, 17, 135, 136, 145, 153, 170
fat, iv, v, ix, 2, 3, 4, 5, 6, 7, 8, 9, 11, 13, 14, 15, 16, 17, 18, 19, 20, 22, 23, 24, 25, 26, 28, 32, 34, 39, 41, 45, 46, 50, 51, 52, 54, 55, 56, 57, 58, 62, 63, 64, 67, 68, 70, 72, 73, 74, 75, 77, 80, 85, 89, 94, 95, 96, 98, 104, 108, 109, 110, 113, 115, 117, 118, 120, 123, 126, 127, 131, 133, 134, 135, 136, 138, 141, 142, 143, 144, 146, 147, 149, 150, 154, 158, 159, 160, 161, 163, 165, 167
fibre, 11, 14, 19, 20, 24, 25, 31, 34, 36, 37, 41, 42, 43, 44, 56, 58, 67, 68, 69, 70, 75, 76, 104, 107, 108, 109, 129, 138, 161, 166, 170
flavonoids, 21, 42, 62, 63, 67, 88, 97, 120
flax, 3, 41, 42, 44, 115
flaxseed, iv, v, ix, 41, 42, 43, 44, 115, 118, 120, 123, 126, 127, 131, 147, 153, 155, 156, 161
food, iv, ix, 1, 4, 5, 7, 8, 9, 10, 11, 12, 14, 16, 17, 24, 25, 26, 36, 39, 40, 44, 47, 51, 52, 53, 54, 56, 57, 58, 59, 61, 65, 66, 69, 70, 72, 73, 74, 77, 78, 80, 82, 86, 87, 89, 91, 92, 95, 96, 104, 111, 115, 117, 118, 119, 120, 125, 126, 128, 129, 130, 131, 132, 133, 135, 136, 137, 138, 139, 140, 141, 142, 143, 144, 145, 146, 147, 148, 150, 151, 153, 155, 156, 157, 158, 159, 160, 161, 162, 163, 164, 165, 166, 167, 168, 169, 170
forskolin (an extract from *Coleous forskohlii*), 97, 119, 120
fucoxanthin, 97, 120

G

Garcinia cambogia (*Garcinia gummi-gutta*), iv, v, ix, 3, 45, 46, 47, 99, 107, 110, 118, 119, 120, 123, 132, 139, 143, 146, 158, 160
Gardenia jasminoides (Cape jasmine), 100
genes, 9, 10, 11, 17, 22, 32, 151
ginger, iv, v, ix, 3, 48, 49, 50, 51, 52, 101, 108, 110, 118, 120, 123, 126, 132, 134, 138, 141, 146, 147, 154, 160, 162, 163, 166
Ginkgo biloba (gingko - the maidenhair tree), 100
ginseng (*Panax spp.*), 97, 98, 100, 120
glucose, 9, 21, 27, 31, 39, 43, 45, 56, 59, 60, 67, 78, 79, 80, 85, 91, 94, 125, 136, 139, 142, 144, 145, 154, 156, 158, 160, 161, 163, 164, 168, 169
Glycine hispida (soybean), 100
Glycine max, 97, 100, 119
Glycyrrhiza uralensis (Chinese liquorice), 100
grapefruit (*Citrus paradisi*), 97, 120, 133
grapes, 87, 110, 111, 114, 115, 120
Griffonia simplicifolia (Bandeiraea simplicifolia Benth), 100
Griffonia simplicifolia (Bandeiraea simplicifolia Benth.), 100
Gymnema sylvestre (Gurmar), 100, 110

H

healthy lifestyle, iv, ix, 14, 15, 17, 18, 19, 123
heat, 5, 9, 10, 11, 17, 18, 20, 32, 50, 71, 73, 86, 89, 96, 108, 113, 120
hesperidin, 97, 98, 109, 111, 120, 149
Hibiscus sabdaroffa, 97, 114, 115, 119, 120
Hoodia gordonii, iv, ix, 52, 53, 55, 119, 123, 129, 146, 160, 161, 165, 169
hormone, 8, 13, 32, 72, 155
hunger, 2, 7, 8, 9, 11, 13, 14, 20, 22, 32, 46, 59, 73, 108, 120
hunger centres, 9, 20, 108

I

Ilex paraguariensis (Yerba Maté), vi, 3, 93, 94, 95, 96, 100, 103, 107, 108, 118, 120, 126, 131, 133, 136, 142
inflammations, 1, 25, 42, 63, 79
Irvingia gabonensis, iv, vi, ix, 3, 55, 56, 57, 58, 89, 109, 110, 118, 120, 123, 125, 135, 137, 143, 148, 150, 151, 152, 158, 163, 170

K

konjac/glucomannan, iv, ix, 3, 123

L

Lagerstroemia speciosa, 97, 120
lemon, 114, 115, 118, 120
lifestyle, iv, ix, 9, 14, 15, 16, 17, 18, 19, 30, 116, 123, 136, 172
Ligularia fischeri (gomchwi or Fischers ragwort), 100
Limonia acidissima (wood-apple), 100
linolenic acid, 41, 42, 120, 170
lipid, 3, 5, 6, 8, 13, 26, 32, 43, 46, 50, 63, 69, 77, 78, 80, 81, 86, 91, 95, 96, 98, 101, 114, 128, 136, 138, 139, 145, 147, 148, 150, 154, 159, 160, 161, 162, 163, 164, 166, 169, 171
liquorice (*Glycyrrhiza glabra*), 97, 100, 119
Lithospermum erythrorhizon (purple gromwell – redroot lithospermum), 101
Lonicera caerulea (sweetberry honeysuckle), 100

Index

lutein, 97, 120
lutein and fucoxanthin,, 97

M

Magnolia officinalis (houpu magnolia or magnolia-bark), 100, 168
Malus hupehensis (tea crabapple), 100
Malus hupehensis (Tea Crabapple), 100
Malus prunifolia (plum-leaved apple), 100
Malva parviflora (cheeseweed), 100
Malva parviflora (Cheeseweed), 100
mechanisms, iv, ix, 3, 7, 9, 10, 14, 17, 21, 28, 46, 50, 51, 52, 53, 55, 59, 72, 80, 85, 95, 97, 105, 108, 114, 117, 123, 127, 134, 138, 145, 149, 151, 153, 154, 162, 164, 168
microbiota, 7, 11, 12, 20, 25, 28, 37, 38, 39, 42, 58, 67, 69, 76, 77, 78, 80, 84, 86, 91, 92, 94, 108, 129, 142, 155, 165
momordica (*Momordica charantia*), 97, 115, 120
Momordica charantia, 97, 115, 120
monosaccharides, 5, 11, 19, 107
Moringa olifera, 97, 120
mormodica (*Momordica charantia*), 97, 115, 120
Morus alba (white mulberry), 61, 62, 63, 64, 65, 66, 100, 110, 132, 139, 146, 148, 168, 169
Morusaustrails poir (mulberry), iv, vi, ix, 3, 61, 62, 63, 64, 65, 66, 100, 107, 108, 110, 118, 120, 123, 139, 144, 146, 163, 167, 168, 169, 170, 173
myths, vi, 3, 15, 113, 114, 123, 169

N

naringin, 97, 120
Nelumbo nucifera Gaertn (Indian lotus), 100
neuromediators, 7, 8, 9, 71

O

oat, iv, vi, ix, 3, 66, 67, 68, 69, 70, 118, 119, 123, 129, 137, 141, 144
orange (*Citrus sinensis*), 45, 98, 119, 120, 133, 156
Origanum dayi (oregano), 100
Oroxylum indicum (oroxylum – Indian trumpet flower), 100
oxidation, 11, 13, 20, 22, 32, 50, 51, 56, 64, 73, 82, 83, 86, 88, 95, 96, 104, 108, 126, 141, 167

P

Panax ginseng (Asian ginseng), 100
Panax japonicus (Japanese ginseng), 100
Panax quinquefolium (American ginseng), 100
Paullinia cupana (guarana), 94, 100, 110
peanuts, 114, 115, 118, 120
peony (*Penia suffruticosa*), 97, 115, 120
Peucedanum japonicum Thunb (coastal hog fennel), 100
Phaseolus vulgaris (common bean), 97, 100, 110, 119
physical activity, 17, 18, 19, 22, 64, 116
pine extract, 97
pineapple, 110, 111, 114, 118, 120
Platycodon grandiflorum (Chinese bellflower), 100
plum, iv, vi, ix, 3, 75, 76, 77, 78, 100, 107, 108, 110, 118, 120, 123, 127, 132, 149, 150, 151, 156, 165, 171
polysaccharides, 5, 11, 14, 19, 24, 62, 63, 107, 139
pomegranate, 100, 110, 114, 115, 118, 120
pomelo, 114, 118, 120, 171
probiotic, 69, 159
proteins, 4, 11, 14, 15, 18, 24, 28, 34, 56, 58, 59, 61, 62, 68, 69, 168

Prunus salicina (Japanese plum), 75, 77, 100, 132, 140, 151
Psidium guajava (common guava), 100
Punica granatum (pomegranate), 100, 110, 114, 115, 118, 120

R

Radix Platycodi (root of Chinese bellflower), 100
Rhizoma coptidis (coptidis – huanglian), 100
Rhus coriaria (Sicilian sumac – tanner's sumach), 100
rosella – red sorrel (*Hibiscus sabdaroffa*), 97, 114, 115, 119, 120
rosemary (*Rosmarinus officinalis*), 100, 114, 115, 118, 120

S

Salacia reticulata (Kothala himbuktu – Salacia), 97, 101, 120
Salicornia europaea (glasswort), 101
Salix matsudana (Chinese willow), 101
Salvia officinalis (sage), 101, 110
Sapindus rarak (sapindus – lerak or klerek), 101
satiety, 7, 8, 9, 19, 20, 22, 35, 39, 57, 69, 77, 80, 97, 105, 108, 126, 136, 137, 139, 146, 147, 159
Sesamum indicum, 97, 120
Seville orange (*Citrus aurantium*), 97, 119
skipping breakfast, 16, 115, 137, 149
smoking, 18
Solanum tuberosum (potato), 18, 101
soy (*Glycine max*), 97, 100, 114, 119, 126
St John's-wort (*Hypericum perforatum*), 114
Stevia rebaudiana, iv, vi, ix, 78, 123, 126, 131, 135, 144, 145, 149, 157, 158

stress, 7, 8, 21, 45, 49, 56, 62, 71, 76, 84, 140, 141, 146, 150, 164
sweetness, 20, 78, 80, 108, 131
Swertia chirayita (Swertia), 101
Swietenia mahogani (American mahogany), 101

T

tangerine, 114, 118, 120
tea, iv, vi, ix, 3, 25, 62, 65, 66, 82, 83, 84, 85, 86, 87, 93, 96, 99, 100, 103, 104, 107, 108, 110, 118, 119, 123, 128, 129, 130, 131, 140, 141, 142, 144, 148, 153, 155, 158, 162, 163, 164, 165, 166, 167, 168
temperature, 7, 9, 71, 83, 104
Bos indicus (humped cattle - zebu, 99
triacylglycerols, 6, 20, 22, 42, 46, 59, 85, 107
Tripterygium wilfordii (thunder god vine), 101

V

Vaccinium ashei (rabbiteye blueberry), 101
veld grape, vi, 3, 87, 118, 120
vitamins, 6, 21, 24, 34, 36, 42, 43, 48, 58, 59, 60, 61, 66, 67, 68, 75, 77, 110, 173
Vitis vinifera (grape vine), 101

W

waist to hip ratio, 6
Wasabia japonica Matsum (wasabi), 101
water, 4, 6, 15, 35, 37, 41, 44, 58, 60, 93, 104, 114, 128, 132, 157
wholegrain bread, 114, 118, 120

Y

Yacón, vi, 3, 90, 91, 92, 108, 128, 130
Yacon and ginger, iv, ix, 123

Z

Zingiber officinale (ginger), iv, v, ix, 3, 48, 49, 50, 51, 52, 101, 108, 110, 118, 120, 123, 126, 132, 134, 138, 141, 146, 147, 154, 160, 162, 163, 166